NATURAL M

for Allergies

....

The Best Alternative Methods for Quick Relief

....

- *Hay fever*
- *Problem foods*
- *Skin rashes, itching*
- *. . . and other symptoms*

GLENN S. ROTHFELD, M.D.

AND SUZANNE LeVERT

Rodale Press, Inc.
Emmaus, Pennsylvania

This book is intended as a reference volume only, not as a medical manual. The information given here is designed to help you make informed decisions about your health. It is not intended as a substitute for any treatment that may have been prescribed by your doctor. If you suspect that you have a medical problem, we urge you to seek competent medical help.

Library of Congress Cataloging-in-Publication Data

Rothfeld, Glenn.
    Natural medicine for allergies : the best alternative methods for quick relief / Glenn S. Rothfeld and Suzanne LeVert.
        p.   cm.
    Includes index.
    ISBN 0–87596–286–6 paperback
      1. Allergy—Alternative treatment. I. LeVert, Suzanne. II. Title.
RC584.R686   1997
616.97'06—dc20   96–2738

Distributed in the book trade by St. Martin's Press

2 4 6 8 10 9 7 5 3 1 paperback

OUR PURPOSE

*"We inspire and enable people to improve
their lives and the world around them."*

Dedication

....

To Magi for her endless love and support,

and to my sons Jedidiah and Eli,

who are brimming with life.

G. S. R.

Acknowledgments

....

I would like to thank Madeleine Morel, Barbara

Lowenstein, and Rodale Press for their help in hatching

and shepherding this idea; AMR'TA, makers of IBIS,

an extraordinary data base of natural medicine;

Ben Benjamin, Catherine LeBlanc, Dr. Daren Fan,

Dr. Richard Glickman-Simon, Lori Grace,

Nancy Lipman, and others who helped me with their

comments and encouragement. I am also grateful

to the many patients who brought me ideas and inspired

me with their own journeys toward better health.

Contents

CHAPTER 1

Allergies and Alternative Medicine **1**

CHAPTER 2

A Medical Overview **17**

CHAPTER 3

Choosing an Alternative **39**

CHAPTER 4

*Understanding Food Allergies
and Dietary Influences* **49**

CHAPTER 5

Acupuncture and Chinese Medicine **67**

CHAPTER 6

Medicine from India **81**

CHAPTER 7

Herbal Medicine at Work **95**

CHAPTER 8

*Spinal and Cranial Manipulation:
Chiropractic and Osteopathy* **107**

CHAPTER 9

Homeopathy and Allergies **117**

CHAPTER 10

Meditation: Re-establishing Internal Balance **125**

CHAPTER 11

Exercising for Health and Fitness **135**

CHAPTER 12

Healing Touch: Bodywork and Massage **149**

CHAPTER 13

Developing an Alternative Plan **159**

Natural Resources **174**

Words and Terms to Remember **188**

Index **194**

About the Authors **202**

"The physician

is only nature's

assistant."

Galen

Allergies and Alternative Medicine

1

*D*oes a waft of goldenrod trigger sneezing fits every spring? Are your eyes set ablaze whenever you cuddle with your best friend's cat? Or are you among those people who become irritable, nauseous, or even depressed and confused after eating certain foods?

If you've answered yes to any of these questions, you're certainly not alone. In fact, about one in every five Americans—roughly 46 million men, women, and children—suffer from allergies. At least 25 million have hay fever or allergic rhinitis, about 9 million have asthma, and another 12 million or more have a variety of allergic disorders triggered by various environmental or food substances. We'll explore in this book is why allergies are so common today and how you can modify your environment and dietary habits in order to reduce your risk of developing or exacerbating allergies and sensitivities.

The substances that can cause an allergic reaction are too numerous to count. They include pollen, plant sap, dust, mold, food, animal hair, insect venom, medication, cosmetics, and even environmental changes, like a burst of cold air or excess humidity. In essence, an allergy occurs when the body's defense system, called the immune system, does not work properly. An allergy exists when the immune system, whose purpose is to defend the body against harmful invaders, unleashes a response against a substance normally considered quite benign. In other words, your body treats pollen like a deadly enemy that must be eliminated at all costs. The symptoms of such an allergy—watery eyes, wheezing, itchy skin, etc.—represent the body's efforts to rid itself of the offending substance.

If you suffer from allergies, it's likely that you've spent a good part of your life frustrated. You may even have to face a certain amount of fear. Will the host at tonight's dinner party serve something that will set off an attack? If you take an antihistamine before the party, will you be sleepy and inattentive? Will this ever end? Unfortunately, experiencing these emotions may set up a vicious cycle, since anxiety itself can cause an allergy to flare up or worsen. Indeed we now know that excess emotional (or physical) stress may disrupt and undermine the immune system, leaving us more vulnerable not only to allergies but to a host of other conditions as well. In addition, more and more research indicates that allergens—substances that cause allergic reactions—affect our spirits and moods just as dramatically as they do our respiratory or dermatological systems. As Chapter 10 explains, learning to refocus and relax your mind and spirit should become an important part of your allergy treatment plan.

The truth is, you may very well have to cope with your body's sensitivities to certain substances for the rest of your life. We'll show you ways to make that reality more manageable, provide tips to make your day-to-day life more comfortable, and offer you healthier options to the pharmaceutical merry-go-round you've probably been on for some time.

You're probably looking for less expensive and less uncomfortable ways to solve your allergy problems. You may also be searching for a way to cope with some of the underlying reasons why your body isn't working the way it should. Fortunately, there are many options available to help you accomplish both of these related goals. Later in this chapter, you'll learn more about the different alternative techniques and philosophies of health and healing that may help you better cope with your allergies. First, however, let's take a closer look at some of the challenges you face as an allergy sufferer.

The Challenge of Chronic Illness

Most Americans tend to assume that doctors can repair all things medical with drugs, surgery, or other quick fixes. If our arteries are clogged with fat, we want to bust the plaque out with a balloon or reroute blood through a bypass instead of changing our diet and exercise habits. If our immune systems overreact—as they do during an allergic reaction—we'd rather take a pill or suffer through allergy shots rather than attempt to correct the underlying imbalance. Indeed, we remain stubbornly (and, in the end, counterproductively) distanced from the intricate nature and quality of health and healing. Unfortunately, this distancing often leaves us frustrated and still unwell even after treatment. Why? Although drugs and surgery may be lifesavers in certain circumstances—when raging bacterial infections take hold or heart attacks or accidents occur—modern medicine remains stymied by conditions of a systemic and/or chronic nature. And allergies certainly fall into that category.

Within the modern Western medical tradition, physicians and researchers often divide health problems into those considered *acute* and those considered *chronic*. Acute health problems generally begin abruptly and have a single, readily identifiable cause. These conditions usually respond well and quickly to specific treatments, such as medication or surgery. When treatment succeeds in eliminating the symptoms and effects of the acute illness, doctors consider patients "cured," or brought back to a normal state of health.

Chronic conditions, on the other hand, tend to start slowly, progress slowly, and endure over several years, even over an entire lifetime. Sometimes, doctors find it difficult to even diagnosis a chronic illness, since its symptoms and course may be both subtle and unpredictable. Unlike acute disease, chronic disease often has several possible, coexisting causes, ranging from genetic factors to lifestyle and environmental influences to individual physiological qualitites. Almost by definition, chronic illnesses have no "cure," no simple solution.

All around us, we see evidence of the failure of modern medicine to grapple with this type of condition. Currently, we are a nation of chronically ill—allergies, arthritis, heart disease, osteoporosis, and obesity remain rampant in the population. So far, we have failed to find effective medical techniques for treating these health problems. The "quick-fix" approach will simply not succeed; instead, we should accept the slower but steadier methods of bringing our bodies back to health as prescribed by the natural schools of medicine described in this book. The foods we eat, the exercise we get, the air we breathe, the cycles of nature, and our own unique physiologies are among the keys to finding long-lasting solutions to chronic conditions like allergies and to achieving physical and emotional health.

Without question, people with allergies are among those in most need of such solutions. You not only must cope with the symptoms of your particular allergy—skin rashes, headaches, and respiratory distress, among others—but must also deal with the side effects of having a chronic illness. Indeed, the long-term nature of most allergies places enormous pressure on your body and spirit. Here are just a few ways that having allergies (or heart disease, osteoporosis, or any other chronic condition) may affect your health and your life:

Fatigue. Whenever a chronic illness is present, the body is less efficient in its use of energy, in part because the body uses some of this energy to try to heal itself. Thus those with allergies are likely to feel exhausted, weak, and listless—and sometimes these states will last so long that you won't remember what it felt like to be energetic and enthusiastic. In fact, you may not remember what just being normally active feels like.

Shortness of Breath. Shortness of breath occurs whenever the body does not get the oxygen it needs. A lack of oxygen leaves the body feeling sapped and the mind less alert. Lack of oxygen can lead to chronic dizziness and incapacity if not effectively treated. Shortness of breath can occur for many different reasons related to allergy: damage to the air sacs in the lungs, narrowing of the air passages, overproduction of mucus, and general deconditioning of muscles. At the same time, people with all types of allergies—not just those whose respiratory system is directly affected by the allergic response—may experience shortness of breath if they remain inactive too long or feel under constant stress.

Pain. Allergy may cause pain in a variety of ways. Allergies themselves frequently cause pain directly: joints may swell and ache in reaction to an allergen, skin and eyes may itch and burn, the very act of breathing may seem excruciating. More indirectly, muscle aches and pains are common among allergy sufferers for two reasons: if an allergy keeps you from being active, your muscles quickly decondition, leaving them vulnerable to sprains and strains. At the same time, the anxiety and stress engendered by having allergies can themselves cause muscles to tense up, cramp, and ache. Finally, being afraid or depressed about your condition will only enhance the pain you feel from any of the above reasons.

Stress. Stress is a frequent side effect of all chronic illnesses, including allergies. In essence, you experience stress whenever your body attempts to meet any demand made upon it, physical or emotional, pleasant or unpleasant. Usually, if the rest of your body is in balance, you can recover quickly from stress once the demand has been met. However, if stress is present for any length of time, your body begins to adapt—or rather maladapt—to the stress. Chronic high blood pressure, inflammation, muscle tension, and shortness of breath are among the resulting conditions. In Chapter 10, we'll discuss stress and how to cope with it in more depth.

Anger. As you probably already know too well, a life with allergies is one beset by uncertainty and unpredictability. Allergies appear to have snatched the control over your own bodily functions you believed you earned once you grew out of diapers. Depending on the severity or frequency of your condition, you may be left feeling helpless and anxious, especially in the middle of a stubborn flare-up. These emotions, coupled with the frequent disruptions of your daily life, are apt to lead to feelings of anger—anger at the fates, at the doctors, at your own body, at all the environmental toxins polluting the world. Learning to manage that anger is another topic we discuss in Chapter 10.

Depression. Fear and anxiety about the future, constant frustration, and the loss of control over your life and body can lead to a case of chronic depression. No doubt you've already felt at least a few passing waves of disappointment, hopelessness, and dips in your self-esteem because of your allergy problems. In order to return your spirit to its proper, balanced state, you must first solve the physical problems related to your immune system and its dysfunction.

As you'll see in Chapter 2, mainstream medicine now offers few lasting options for treating allergies. The symptoms and causes are too complex and variable, at least so far. Holistic medicine, on the other hand, is remarkably suited to treating a disease like allergy. Its view of health is based on establishing and maintaining internal balance, and on helping the body to maintain its own proper structure and function by providing it with all the nutrients, physical exercise, and emotional support it requires.

The Benefits of Holistic Health Care

In 1992, the National Institutes of Health, the federal government's largest supporter of medical research, announced the establishment of the Office of Alternative Medicine. Its goal remains to explore fresh approaches to such chronic diseases as cancer, AIDS, arthritis, and allergies, for which standard medicine offers limited treatment. In part, the decision to open the office stemmed from the mounting evidence that increasing numbers of Americans seek alternative care every year—with or without their mainstream doctor's sanction—for a whole host of minor and major illnesses. Research indicates that alternative medicine continues to be big business: American consumers spend upward of $15 billion every year on visits to homeopaths, acupuncturists, chiropractors, herbalists, and other holistic practitioners.

Why is there such an interest in alternative theories and practices, especially since most of us have been brought up to expect the "quick fix"? Indeed, to attain health with natural medicine takes time and commitment, especially in this society where the very habits of daily life often conspire to undermine spiritual and physical well-being. Bringing the body into harmony means providing it with the right kind of fuel by eating properly, massaging its organs and tissues through regular exercise, and allowing its internal environment to rest and regenerate in peace through meditation and other relaxation strategies.

On the other hand, there are times when modern medical technology and pharmacology perform lifesaving miracles. Antibiotics fight infections that would otherwise spread through the body too quickly for natural medicine to effectively stop. The surgical removal of cancerous tissue may be necessary to halt the invasion of abnormal cells into essential organs. As someone with allergies, you know how effective—at least in the short term—antihistimines and corticosteroids can be during a severe allergy attack. In Chapter 2 we'll explore in depth some of the ways that modern medicine can and should be used to prevent serious complications from occuring during an allergy attack.

In the meantime, it might help you to think about how the treatment of allergies differs within the alternative and mainstream traditions. Here are just a few of the issues you may want to consider:

HOLISTIC MEDICINE

Provides safer treatment options. Alternative medicine works by helping your body to heal itself. Drugs, on the other hand, work either by taking over the body's functions or by temporarily alleviating itchiness, respiratory distress, or whatever other physical expressions your allergies might take. Your body never fully heals, then, but is merely compelled to operate through the physiological crisis. In addition, drugs often have side effects—such as drowsiness and confusion—that alternative therapies such as herbs and relaxation strategies generally avoid.

Focuses on the individual not the condition. Practitioners of natural medicine recognize that every person with an allergy develops the condition under a different set of circumstances. Because there are so many different triggers of allergies, and because there are so many underlying causes of immune system malfunction, no one type of therapy will cure it. Treating your particularly type of allergy or set of sensitivities with alternative medicine involves not a simple prescription or operation, but a comprehensive plan that recognizes your unique emotional, spiritual, and physical makeup.

Involves the whole body. According to most alternative disciplines, the systems and organs involved in the allergic response do not exist in isolation from the rest of the body. Nor do they remain unaffected by emotions, thoughts, or external stressors. The practitioner of Chinese medicine, the herbalist, or the chiropractor looks at the whole person from head to toe, physically and emotionally, when treating any condition, including allergy. To treat your case of hay fever, for example, may involve far more than your respiratory system. It may very well extend to the emotional level and how you feel about yourself.

Validates the emotional component of health. Although it seems clear that emotional stress and upheavals have a direct impact on the body's ability to function, Western medicine has resisted using this knowledge to prevent or treat disease. Not only does natural medicine acknowledge the integral role your emotions play in maintaining health, but its traditions use these factors in creating a comprehensive treatment plan for virtually every disease and condition. This mind/body approach is especially useful in healing your immune system. There have been several studies showing that the more hope you feel and the more positive energy you have, the more immune system cells you produce and the better your immune system performs. Although this information has not yet been applied to the treatment of allergies, there is every reason to believe that bringing your emotional and spiritual life into balance will leave you better able to cope with your allergies and maybe even better able to fight them off.

Helps to prevent as well as treat. Establishing and maintaining the body's natural, balanced state is the goal of natural medicine, not just treating one isolated condition or problem. By bringing your body back into balance in order to help alleviate your allergies, you may well be helping to strengthen your body in many other ways as well. If you visit a homeopath for treatment of your allergies, for instance, you may find that the treatment alleviates another recurrent health problem too, such as an arthritic knee or an acidic stomach. This is because the remedies applied work on many different levels and systems throughout the body. In addition, the more balanced and healthy your body is, the less vulnerable it is to developing other conditions and diseases.

Helps you find the natural rhythm of health. Your body is a remarkable vessel of biochemical actions and reactions that allow you to breathe, to digest your food, to dream, and to hope. Natural approaches to health and healing allow your body to work as nature intended, without the need for man-made and potentially side-effect-ridden interventions. Furthermore, alternative therapies attempt to create a healthier relationship between your body and the natural environment. It's likely that you'll be encouraged to be outside more, to take walks, to meditate about your place in the universe and within your community as part of your overall treatment. In that way, you're likely to develop a new, stronger bond with the world around you.

For these reasons, you may decide to join the millions of Americans now using one or more natural remedies to treat their allergies and to restore internal harmony and balance within their bodies. This book is intended to help you sort through the many alternative approaches available and evaluate which ones may work best for your particular situation.

Nine Natural Approaches
to Treating Allergies

Before we outline the various approaches covered in this book, we must stress the importance of visiting a mainstream physician for an evaluation of your condition. By taking advantage of mainstream diagnostic procedures, you'll be able to rule out serious medical problems such as infections, more serious autoimmune diseases, and other conditions that may be at the root of your symptoms—and which may require a more immediate mainstream treatment to resolve.

On the other hand, if you're like most people with allergy, you've already discovered the limitations of modern medicine when it comes to treating your condition. The good news is that you may well hold the solution within yourself: your own body can heal itself if given the right ingredients and the right environment in which to do so.

Outlined below are nine different types of alternative therapy that are appropriate for treating allergies. In many ways, they are all inter-related, having in common the aspects of balance and self-healing. Some of them, such as herbal medicine and Chinese medicine, offer complete philosophies of health and comprehensive strategies for treating allergies. Others, such as exercise and bodywork, will help you to establish healthier physical patterns and habits, allowing you to meet the challenges of your allergies with more self-confidence and spiritual strength. We'll introduce you to their basic theories and techniques in hopes that, should one or more of them interest you, you'll take the time to explore them more thoroughly by reading other books and visiting qualified practitioners.

UNDERSTANDING FOOD ALLERGIES AND
DIETARY INFLUENCES

Chapter 4 discusses the connection between what you eat and how you feel. Food allergies can cause several types of direct reactions, including nausea, diarrhea, and vomiting as well as rashes, respiratory dysfunction, headaches, and dizziness, among others. In addition, a food allergy may be so subtle as to go unrecognized, yet disrupt the entire immune system, thus leaving the body vulnerable to developing allergies to other foods and substances. An allergy to yeast is an example. Also, a yeast overgrowth could become a problem due to an illness or immune system failure. Not only does too much yeast itself cause gastrointestinal discomfort, it also triggers the immune system into hyperactivity. In Chapter 4 we'll discuss these problems—and some solutions—in depth, as well as show you ways to improve your diet to boost your immune system.

ACUPUNCTURE AND CHINESE MEDICINE

Stemming from a centuries-old tradition, Chinese medicine and acupuncture view health not only as the absence of disease, but also as the existence of a balanced and harmonious internal environment. It is based on the view that humanity is part of a larger creation—the universe itself—and is thus subject to the same laws that govern the stars, the soil, and the sea. Harmony and health, within the body and within the universe, depend on the careful balance of two opposing forces of nature called yin and yang. Furthermore, an energy called qi (pronounced "chee") permeates the entire universe and is the source of life and strength for all living matter.

In Chinese medicine, all health care is designed to balance qi and to bring yin and yang into harmony. According to Chinese medical theory, allergies are caused by a deficiency or weakness of qi. If qi is deficient in the lungs, for example, respiratory symptoms like sneezing, dry coughing, and wheezing might result. If qi is deficient in the spleen, it might lead to mucous accumulation, a stuffy nose, and digestive problems. A qi deficiency related to the kidney, on the other hand, might lead to an exhaustion of the immune and nervous system.

A primary method of releasing blocked qi and restoring yin/yang balance is with acupuncture: the use of needles to direct qi to organs or functions of the body or to disperse qi where it is excessive. As we'll discuss in detail in Chapter 5, practitioners of Chinese medicine also use herbal medicine, diet and nutrition, and a form of exercise known as qi-gong.

MEDICINE FROM INDIA

Based on a system developed in India around the fifth century B.C., Ayurveda, like Chinese medicine, considers health within a universal context. Within the human body exists a universal energy or life force called prana. Prana provides every human being with the vitality and endurance to live in harmony with the universe, as well as offers the body the power to heal itself. Balance and harmony within the body are maintained by what is known as the *three doshas*, which are forces of energy that act upon body substances and organs. The goal of Ayurvedic medicine is to keep the three doshas balanced so that the body can function in health. When they are out of balance, disease and disorder results. Allergy, for instance, is most often associated with the dosha known as "kapha," which is related to the season of winter, when the respiratory system tends to be more vulnerable to congestion.

In Chapter 6, you'll see how an Ayurvedic practitioner might consider your condition and how he or she might treat your allergies according to Ayurvedic principles. Such treatment includes diet, yoga, herbs, and meditation exercises.

HERBAL MEDICINE AT WORK

Herbal medicine and its cousin aromatherapy use plants, herbs, and other natural substances—including venom extracted from honeybees—to stimulate the body to return to the state of internal balance we call health. Though herbs are medicines, they tend to be much safer than chemical drugs for a variety of reasons. They are less potent, are more recognizable to the body as natural substances, and are usually used in combinations and potencies that minimize side effects. Herbal therapy is highly individualized, and herbal prescriptions are not based on a diagnosis of a specific disease—such as allergies—but rather on the needs of each person based on his or her particular symptoms. In other words, an herbalist or aromatherapist may well treat your case of hay fever in a completely different way than he or she would another person with the very same medical diagnosis.

Essential oils used in aromatherapy exude fragrances that have been used as components of medical treatment for centuries. Derived from plants, each oil has its own distinct odor that stimulates an array of emotional and psychological responses that, in turn, work with certain physical reactions to help heal the body. Aromatherapists maintain that each plant has its own set of specific healing qualities, based upon where it was grown and under what conditions. Chapter 7 discusses how you can use herbs and oils to treat your allergies. In general, herbs are used to alleviate symptoms as well as to strengthen the immune system.

SPINAL AND CRANIAL MANIPULATION

Chapter 8 introduces you to two related branches of alternative medicine: chiropractic and osteopathy. According to the theory behind chiropractic therapy, the spine is the well from which the body's innate intelligence springs. If the vertebrae of the spine are not properly aligned, this intelligence cannot flow to other parts of the body to assure their proper functioning. Realigning the spine can thus alleviate both the symptoms and the underlying causes of allergies of all kinds—those that affect the skin, the respiratory system, the gastrointestinal tract, and the central nervous system.

Osteopathy is another system that involves adjusting the body in order to improve its overall function and health. Osteopaths receive standard physician training (their degree, doctor of osteopathy, is equivalent to that of a medical doctor), but their education also includes courses on how to adjust the spine and other skeletal structures in order to return the body to a state of internal balance. Cranial osteopathy, which concentrates on realigning the joints of the skull, offers special benefit to those people who suffer from respiratory distress due to allergies.

HOMEOPATHY AND ALLERGIES

Chapter 9 explores homeopathy and its relationship to allergies. A system of medicine that attempts to harness the body's own healing power to fight disease and maintain health, homeopathy was developed by a nineteenth-century German scientist named Samuel Hahnemann. It is based on the principle that "like cures like," that medications should be given not to counteract the symptoms of illness, as they are in mainstream medicine, but rather to stimulate the body to cure itself. Because allergies involve the overstimulation of the immune system, homeopathic remedies tend to concentrate on reversing this process.

MEDITATION: RE-ESTABLISHING INTERNAL BALANCE

Chapter 10 describes the relationship between stress and the development or exacerbation of allergies. We will guide you through several methods of meditation and relaxation designed to help you recognize and then release your own particular brand of negative stress. These methods include progressive relaxation, guided imagery, and biofeedback among others.

EXERCISING FOR HEALTH AND FITNESS

As admonitions about the importance of exercise continue to dominate the headlines of health magazines, Americans—and American doctors—are finally beginning to accept that regular exercise is essential to health. Exercise helps the intestines digest food more effectively, your brain stay alert and stimulated, and your respiratory system function at its optimal level.

Your body needs to move in order for you to stay well. Your brain, your heart, your lungs, your skin, your internal organs, your muscles, all need the increased blood flow and stimulation that exercise provides. Moving your body also helps to transport waste products—including potential allergens—from every cell in your body. In Chapter 11, we'll show you how to make exercise a regular part of your life in order to condition your whole body safely and effectively.

HEALING TOUCH: BODYWORK AND MASSAGE

In Chapter 12, you'll read about several different movement awareness and massage therapies, such as the Alexander technique and Rolfing, which attempt to both alleviate current stress and tension and realign the body to help establish balance, confidence, and self-awareness. Healing through touch has been a part of healing traditions around the world for centuries, and you may well find relief from your allergy symptoms through one or more of these methods. Some of these techniques require the involvement of a trained professional; others you can learn to do on your own with some guidance.

Following these chapters on the basics of alternative medicine, Chapter 13 raises and answers some of the most common questions about allergies and the various therapies offered here to treat it. Finally, we provide you with a host of resources, including organizations, associations, and books, that will guide you should you choose to further explore any or all of the methods outlined in this book.

In the meantime, however, the next chapter provides you with an understanding of allergies from a physiological perspective. Chapter 2 explains exactly what happens in your body, and why, when an allergic reaction occurs.

"Disease is the retribution of outraged Nature."

Hosea Ballou

A Medical Overview

$\mathcal{T}$he healthy human body is a virtual citadel—a self-contained structure highly protected against harmful invaders from the outside world. It has a protective wall (the skin), a first line of defense (the tiny hairs of the nose, certain enzymes in the mouth's saliva), and a complex and organized army patrolling the internal environment. When functioning as it should, this defense organization allows the body's population of organs, tissues, and fluids to flourish in harmony. When we're healthy, digestion, respiration, imagination, emotion, and movement all take place unhindered, largely without conscious thought, and all under the careful "watch" of the army of immune system cells. Constantly streaming through lymph and blood vessels throughout the body, immune cells attempt to ensure that outside enemies do not upset the careful balance within.

And today, it seems as if there are more and more enemies ready to invade and disrupt. Not only do we have to guard against natural organisms that have always been present, such as viruses, bacteria, and fungi, but also against a whole host of synthetic pollutants in the air, in the soil, in our food, even in our medicines. Although the immune system has successfully evolved and adapted to myriad enemies and stresses, scientists now believe that many of us suffer from allergies because the sheer number of substances—harmful and good—entering our systems every day simply overwhelms our capacity to identify and absorb them. Nevertheless, the body's defense system remains remarkably effective and adept. Before we explore exactly how and why it may go wrong to cause the body to develop an allergy, let's take a look at a healthy immune system at work.

The Immune System at Work

The word immunity comes from the Latin word *immunitas*, which in ancient Rome meant the release of an individual from an obligation to serve the state. Today, we use the word immunity in a similar way. For instance, when a known criminal testifies in court in exchange for his own freedom, we say he is "immune" from prosecution. To be immune from a disease means that you are, in a way, "exempt" from getting it. Your body has specific mechanisms to protect you against it.

The immune system's special characteristic is the ability to recognize other cells in the body. It can tell the differences between harmful microbes, cancer cells, and the body's own healthy cells. Put very simply, it's as if each cell wears a uniform and the patrolling guards— white blood cells known as lymphocytes—can distinguish one uniform from another, friend or foe.

When a cell provokes a response from the immune system—that is, when lymphocytes recognize an enemy "uniform"—that cell is called an antigen. Viruses, bacteria, protozoa, and fungi are antigens because they provoke an immune system response once they enter the body. Transplanted tissues and organs, and sometimes our own cells (if they are cancer cells), are also antigens, because lymphocytes do not recognize them as part of the body. Lymphocytes recognize antigens as enemies and then begin a process of defense against them.

In essence, an allergy is caused by a "misfiring" of this defense system. For reasons as yet poorly understood, immune system cells mistakenly identify harmless substances—like cat dander or pollen—as antigens and mount an attack against them. (When harmless antigens cause an immune system response, the antigens are called "allergens.") The symptoms of allergies, including wheezing, sneezing, and skin rashes, represent the outward signs of your body's attempt to rid itself of what it perceives to be harmful enemies.

As the following section reveals, the process of defense mounted by the immune system is remarkably complicated and—when functioning properly—quite effective at protecting our bodies from harm. Later in this chapter, we'll explore how and why allergic responses occur. In the meantime, let's take a look at the way your body's defense system is *supposed* to function.

UNDERSTANDING THE IMMUNE RESPONSE

There are two main classes of immune system cells, T cells and B cells, each of which responds in a different way to threats from antigens. T cells have a molecular code on their surface that directly corresponds to specific antigens, which means that T cells can destroy enemy cells on contact. T cells also work with other immune system cells to either stimulate activity or suppress immune function.

B cells, on the other hand, do not kill antigens directly, but instead produce a type of immune system cell called an antibody or immunoglobulin. Antibodies are the primary defense cells against most types of antigens. They are produced when a B cell comes into contact with an antigen (or allergen) that it recognizes as an enemy. Once the antigen or allergen locks onto the B cell, the B cell then rapidly and repeatedly divides, creating hundred of new cells (called plasma cells) that release antibodies in massive amounts.

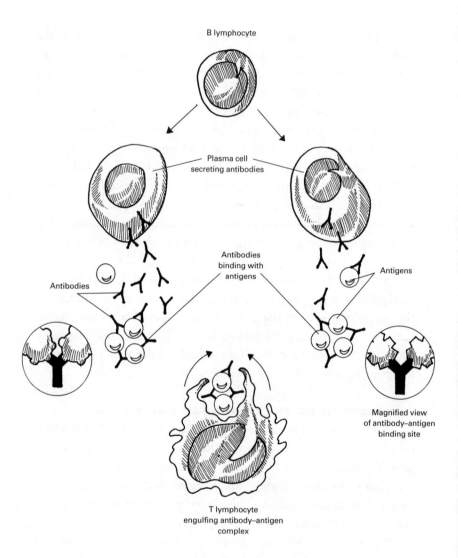

Allergic Reactions

*An allergic reaction takes place on a cellular level.
When an allergen enters the body, it stimulates the production
of cells called B lymphocytes. B lymphocytes, in turn,
stimulate the production of substances called antibodies. Antibodies
bind with the allergens, leading to their destruction.*

Antibodies attempt to render antigens harmless in a number of different ways. If the antigen produces a toxin, for instance, the antibody may be able to directly neutralize the harmful substance. Or antibodies can force enemy microbes together into a clump, allowing other immune system cells to rapidly destroy them. After the crisis that stimulated their release is over, antibodies circulate in the body for some time, then die off. At the same time that activated B cells produce antibodies, however, they also produce what are called *memory cells*. Memory cells, as their name implies, can immediately recognize the specific antigen that first provoked their production—whether it's a cold virus or an allergen like a piece of cat dander. When that antigen reenters the body, memory cells quickly stimulate an immune system reaction. That's why it sometimes takes only moments after you come into contact with pollen or cat dander for your eyes to start to water or your bronchial tubes to constrict: your immune system cells immediately recognize—however mistakenly—the perceived enemy and mount a quick response to it.

UNDERSTANDING THE ALLERGIC RESPONSE

Antibodies are also known as immunoglobulins or Igs. Scientists have identified five major classes of immunoglobulins, each of which acts in a slightly different way against foreign invaders. Let's take a quick look at each subset of Igs and then concentrate on the one type that scientists believe to be responsible for the majority of the most common allergies, immunoglobulin E, IgE. It is the way that IgE acts in the body that causes allergic symptoms to occur.

IgM is the largest immunoglobulin in structure and the first antibody the body makes when challenged by an antigen. It acts to increase production of other types of immunoglobulins.

IgA is found in all secretions of the body and is the major antibody in the mucous membrane (mucosa) of the intestines and the bronchi, in saliva, and in tears. By combining with the protein in mucosa, it is able to defend body surfaces against invading microorganisms. It also works to identify foreign substances and then trigger the immune response to them.

IgD is a specialized protein found in small amounts in tissue. Although the precise function of IgD is unknown, scientists discovered that it increases in quantity during allergic reactions to milk, insulin, penicillin, and various toxins.

IgG is perhaps the best known of the immunoglobulins. IgG fights infection from bacteria, fungi, and viruses. Under certain circumstances, a doctor might give you an injection of IgG to protect you against an organism to which you may become or have been exposed. When someone you know has hepatitis, for instance, you may receive a type of IgG injection called gamma globulin so that your body is better prepared to fight against the virus that causes hepatitis in case you've been exposed. IgG molecules also appear to be involved in certain allergic responses, including food allergies. As you'll see in Chapter 4, some food allergy tests target IgG molecules.

IgE is the immunoglobulin considered most involved in allergic reactions. Concentrated in the lung, the skin, and the cells of mucous membranes, it offers the body its prime protection against antigens from the environment.

IgE molecules (and perhaps other immunoglobulins) react to otherwise benign substances (called allergens) like pollen, cat dander, and certain foods. They act aggressively to rid the body of the offending allergens, and by doing so, create irritating and sometimes painful—even deadly—symptoms and reactions. In people with allergies, the IgE antibodies to their specific allergens exist by the millions.

When antibodies encounter their specific allergen, they immediately trigger the release of certain chemicals called *mediators*. The best known mediator is histamine. Histamine causes the most familiar allergic reactions: released in the nose, eyes, and sinuses, histamine stimulates sneezing, runny nose, and itchy eyes; released in the lungs it causes narrowing and swelling of the lining of the airways and the secretion of mucus; in the skin, rashes and hives; and in the digestive system, cramping and diarrhea. Another circulating white blood cell involved in the immune response is called the eosinophil. When an allergic reaction occurs, the number of eosinophils increases in the blood and in nasal and bronchial secretions. Other mediators include a family of compounds called kinins, which the immune system releases at the same time as histamine. Prostaglandins, leukotrines, and other mediators are released later in the allergic response. Each may cause other types of reactions within the body, including headaches, mood disruptions, and other symptoms.

Occasionally, the entire body will be affected by the allergic response in a condition known as anaphylactic shock. This serious medical crisis involves the sudden narrowing of blood vessels and air passages, causing a slowing of the pulse, breathing difficulty, and often unconsciousness. (Anaphylactic shock and its treatment are discussed later in the chapter.)

Each allergen produces its own set of IgE antibodies. For this reason, a person may be sensitive to cat dander, for example, but be able to tolerate pollen or industrial chemicals quite well. At the same time, it is quite possible for someone to have many different IgE antibodies and thus be sensitive to many allergens.

Although allergy is the most common immune system disorder, there are many others. In fact, all immune system cells must be present and in good working order for you to stay healthy. When even just one type of lymphocyte malfunctions, it may cause widespread problems throughout the body. In some cases, there is a lack of certain immune system cells, a condition called immune deficiency. The disease known as AIDS (acquired immunodeficiency syndrome) involves a virus that targets and destroys T-helper cells. Eventually, the lack of T-helper cells disrupts the entire immune system and leaves the body vulnerable to infectious and other diseases it would otherwise be able to protect itself against. Another type of immune system disorder, called autoimmunity, results in such diseases as rheumatoid arthritis and pernicious anemia. In these cases, the immune system mistakenly identifies the body's own cells as enemies and sets about to destroy them. In certain types of arthritis, for instance, immune system cells attack the body's collagen tissue, which lines the joints and protects the ends of bones from rubbing together. Once collagen is sufficiently deficient, bone tissue can be lost due to friction, and moving the joint can be extremely painful.

As for allergies, it is still unclear what exactly cause the immune system to overreact to certain substances. We do know that the immune system does not work in isolation from the rest of the body. The endocrine system, which produces hormones, and the nervous system, which carries messages to and from the brain and every cell in the body, are particularly integral—in ways as yet poorly understood—to the functioning of the immune system. The adrenal glands, for instance, produce a hormone called adrenaline (also known as epinephrine). Adrenaline has the function of preparing the body for the "fight-or-flight" response by increasing the heart rate and the force of muscular contraction and opening up the bronchial tubes to allow more oxygen into the lungs. In fact, during severe allergy attacks, doctors give injections of adrenaline in order to relax constricted airways and clogged noses and throats. As we'll discuss further in Chapters 8 and 12, chiropractors and bodywork specialists attempt to ensure that the adrenal glands (located atop the kidneys) are able to function properly in order to produce sufficient quantities of adrenaline naturally.

In the meantime, let's take a look at some of the common theories about allergies currently postulated by medical science.

ALLERGIES: CAUSES AND RISK FACTORS

Although scientists know more about the immune system and how it works than ever before—and continue to learn more every day thanks to widespread research relating to the AIDS virus—they still do not fully understand why and how someone develops allergies. Although you now know more about what happens in your body when you come into contact with a substance to which you are allergic, you no doubt still ask: but why do I have allergies? What you're really asking is: why is my immune system so out of whack? What has caused it to become hypervigilant and hypersensitive to benign substances like ragweed or milk or perfume? Unfortunately, so far, no one knows the answers to those questions. But some of the theories about the causes of allergies, and some of the reasons why allergies seem more common today than ever before, include the following:

Genetics. It appears that some of us inherit from our parents a susceptibility to the development of allergies. That is not to say that we directly inherit an allergy to any specific substance. Rather, it seems as if we might inherit some kind of immune system defect or weakness that leaves us more vulnerable to allergies. For instance, we know that someone whose parents suffer from rheumatoid arthritis— a disease caused by a related immune system defect—is at greater risk of developing allergies than someone whose parents do not suffer from any immune system impairments.

Overexposure to Toxins. Many scientists believe that the large amount of pollutants to which we are exposed day after day, year after year—in the air we breathe, the food we eat, the water we drink, even the clothes we wear—so disrupts our immune systems that they become hypersensitive and hyperactive, unable to differentiate between harmful and benign substances.

Overstimulation by Medicines. Another way that the immune system becomes "confused" by overstimulation may well be through the overuse of certain medications, especially antibiotics to treat bacterial infections. Antibiotics have wide-ranging effects on the body—not all of them positive and many of them potentially leading to or exacerbating allergies. It appears that antibiotics disrupt the internal balance of the body by destroying not only harmful bacteria by "friendly" bacteria as well. The bacteria acidophilus, for instance, helps to protect the small intestine and vagina against infection by yeast and, as we'll discuss further, yeast overgrowth can lead to several different kinds of allergies and allergic reactions. Many scientists believe that antibiotic use leads directly to the development of food intolerances and allergies in later life.

Dietary and Nutritional Problems. What you eat and how well you digest your food may have an enormous impact on the way your immune system functions and reacts—or overreacts—to foreign substances. For instance, eating too much of one kind of food, such as wheat or milk, may eventually trigger an allergy not only to that food but to related foods as well. Any nutritional deficiency, including a lack of one or more essential vitamins or minerals, can lead to a general weakness of the immune system, undermining its ability to function properly.

One of the most prevalent nutritional problems related to allergies is the disease known as *candidiasis*, an infection by a yeast organism known as *Candida albicans*. This is a nutritional problem because yeast is found in so many different foods. *Candida* naturally lives within every human body; as long as the immune system keeps it in check, it doesn't cause problems. Should the immune system become disrupted for any reason—because you're taking immunosuppressant drugs to treat another disease or when you're under excess stress, for example—yeast can spread through the body, challenging the immune system and, finally, undermining it. This can lead to the development of sometimes severe and sometimes subtle sensitivities and allergies to a wide range of substances.

Emotional Stress. Although a certain amount of stress is a normal part of our lives, prolonged bouts of stress can lead to a depletion and disruption of the immune system. This leaves the body more vulnerable to any number of illnesses and conditions, including an increased susceptibility to allergies. And here we find ourselves in another vicious cycle: stress may cause or exacerbate allergies, and allergies themselves increase both physical and emotional stress on the body. It is important, then, to control the amount of stress in your life and choose healthy ways to cope with the stress that remains. We'll show how in Chapter 6.

Types of Allergies

There are as many types of allergic reaction as there are allergens and people with allergies. In general, however, allergies are broken down into the following categories: skin allergies (including contact dermatitis, atopic dermatitis, and hives), respiratory allergies (including hay fever/allergic rhinitis, allergies to dust, dander, and mold, and asthma), food allergies, drug allergies, and nonorganic allergies (i.e., allergies to industrial chemicals, pesticides, synthetics, and air pollution). Let's take them one by one.

SKIN ALLERGIES

Most Americans are susceptible to skin allergies or reactions at some point during their lives. Poison ivy and poison oak are the most common culprits, causing itchy, blistering rashes, but almost any substance can cause an allergic reaction in the skin. The most common skin allergies are described below.

Contact Dermatitis (Allergic). An inflammation of the skin caused by contact with an irritant (such as a strong acid or alkali) is called contact dermatitis. Studies show that the six most common causes of the condition are (1) poison ivy, oak, and sumac; (2) paraphenylenediamine, a chemical used in hair and fur dye, leather, rubber, and printing; (3) nickel compounds; (4) rubber compounds; (5) ethylenediamine, a preservative in creams and eye solutions; and (6) dichromates used in textile ink, paints, and leather processing. Some chemicals used in antiperspirants and cosmetics also cause skin rashes, as do certain drugs, such as penicillin, Novocain, and streptomycin.

Generally speaking, contact dermatitis occurs after prolonged exposure to the offending substance. In addition, the irritation caused by the allergy is likely to be localized to wherever the interaction occurs rather than all over the body. If you develop contact dermatitis when you wear a wool sweater, for instance, the rash would appear on your chest, arms, neck and back, but not on your legs or feet. Generally speaking, symptoms occur within two days after exposure, though sensitive people can develop symptoms within a few hours.

Atopic Dermatitis. Also known as eczema, atopic dermatitis most often occurs in babies and children, although it can appear at any time of life. Although atopic dermatitis itself is not an allergy, about a third of all people with the disorder also develop respiratory allergies such as hay fever and asthma.

Atopic dermatitis consists of patches of dry, extremely itchy, thickened skin. It most often affects the skin behind the knees and in the folds of the elbow. Persistent itching is the most prevalent symptom.

Hives. Also known as urticaria, hives are itchy eruptions characterized by raised, reddened, swollen welts. These lesions usually occur in batches, rather than singly, and they may last a few minutes or for several days. They often worsen and/or spread when you scratch them.

Hives can also be accompanied by swelling of certain body parts, like the tongue, lips, and feet. The welts caused by hives may appear in one place on the body and then disappear after a short period of time, only to then reappear in an another place. Feelings of fear, depression, panic, and anxiety often accompany a case of hives.

About one in five people experience hives at one time or another during their lives. Any number of substances or situations can cause hives, from foods to insect bites, to nervousness and stress. Fish, shellfish, and milk are the foods most commonly involved in allergic reactions resulting in hives; penicillin and aspirin are the chief drug offenders; and cat dander, pollen, and insect bites other culprits.

ALLERGY TIP

If you have a food allergy, be sure to read all labels carefully, and don't be deceived by labels that claim the product is "pure," "natural," or "100 percent natural." A careful reading of the fine print may reveal artificial ingredients like colorings, flavorings, and preservatives—any of which may cause an allergic reaction in a susceptible individual.

RESPIRATORY ALLERGIES

Allergies of the respiratory tract most often produce symptoms similar to those of a cold, including congested nasal passages, runny nose, coughing, wheezing, and sneezing. For some people, these symptoms appear only during pollen season, which can extend from early April to November in most areas of the country. For others, symptoms manifest themselves only in the winter when homes and offices are closed to ventilation, causing irritants like dust, molds, mites, and other common airborne allergens to accumulate. Still others experience symptoms whenever they come into contact with furry animals. Although most respiratory allergies represent responses of the immune system to airborne allergens, some can develop in response to foods and chemicals as well.

Allergic Rhinitis and Hay Fever. Although the terms "allergic rhinitis" and "hay fever" are often used interchangeably, there are subtle differences between the two problems. Hay fever is caused by the pollen of certain flowers, which usually are present only in the spring and fall. Hay fever thus tends to be a seasonal condition. Allergic rhinitis, on the other hand, affects susceptible individuals all year long. People with allergic rhinitis may suffer a sensitivity not only to pollen but also to mold, smoke, perfumes, and industrial chemicals, among many other substances. In addition, any number of food substances from milk to wheat to nuts and shellfish can cause hay-feverlike symptoms as well.

At the same time, people with allergic rhinitis and hay fever have a lot in common when it comes to the symptoms with which they suffer, including nasal stuffiness, sneezing, itchy eyes, and postnasal drip. Violent and repeated sneezing is also common. Usually attacks of hay fever and allergic rhinitis last about 15 to 20 minutes and happen several times a day.

Allergies to Mold, Dander, and Dust. Many people are allergic not only to pollen but to other inhaled allegens such as molds, animal dander, and the mites that live in house dust. Molds are found outside during the summer and early winter and are carried by the wind. Common molds include *Alternaria* and *Hormodendrum.* Indoor molds thrive in dark, musty places as well as in upholstered furniture, rugs, beds, stuffed animals, and books. Common indoor molds include *Penicillium, Aspergillus,* and *Rhizopus.*

The tiny microscopic insects that live in dust cause allergic reactions in millions of people. Mites can also be found in furniture, blankets, carpets, and draperies. Finally, animal dander remains one of the most stubborn and troublesome allergens. Contrary to popular belief, it is not the fur or feathers of pets that cause the allergic reactions, but instead it is the dander, the scales shed from the skin, feathers, and fur of animals and birds.

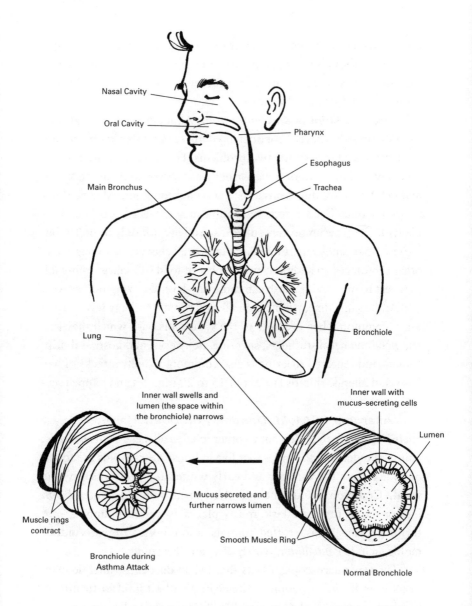

Nasal Cavity

Oral Cavity

Pharynx

Esophagus

Main Bronchus

Trachea

Lung

Bronchiole

Inner wall swells and lumen (the space within the bronchiole) narrows

Inner wall with mucus–secreting cells

Lumen

Mucus secreted and further narrows lumen

Muscle rings contract

Smooth Muscle Ring

Bronchiole during Asthma Attack

Normal Bronchiole

An Asthma Attack

When an asthma attack takes place, the lung's bronchial tubes constrict and become filled with mucus. This results in the wheezing and breathing difficulties experienced during an allergic asthma attack.

Asthma. Characterized by wheezing, tightness in the chest, coughing, and difficulty breathing, asthma is often related to and aggravated by allergies to pollen, mold spores, and other inhaled substances. In addition, allergies to drugs (especially penicillin and aspirin) have been known to cause an asthma attack. For reasons as yet poorly understood, some people have asthma attacks when they exercise, especially during cold weather.

Asthma affects almost 10 million Americans. A majority of those with asthma are children, many of whom outgrow the problem during adolescence, although asthma can develop at any age.

OTHER SYMPTOMS AND REACTIONS

In addition to the more common symptoms described above, an allergy to any kind of substance can result in one or more of the following reactions:

Anaphylactic Shock. The most severe and potentially deadly of allergic reactions, anaphylaxis is most often experienced by people who have a history of allergies and therefore have memory cells ready to provoke an immediate and widespread allergic response as soon as an allergen is detected. Anaphylaxis causes a constriction or narrowing of the airways and the blood vessels, resulting in difficult breathing, rapid pulse, a fall in blood pressure, and even cardiovascular collapse and shock. Anaphylaxis is a critical medical emergency requiring immediate injections of the hormone epinephrine, which opens the airways and blood vessels. It is also treated with oxygen, antihistamines, and steroids, among other medications. People known to have severe reactions to insect bites and other allergens should carry emergency kits containing epinephrine.

Headaches. Any type of headache may be caused by allergic reactions. Certain foods in particular have been implicated as frequent triggers of migraine or migraine-type headaches. Foods containing the substance tyramine (including chocolate and aged cheeses), monosodium glutamate and other food additives, and red wines are frequent culprits. Nonfood triggers include cigarette smoke and other pollutants, pollen, dust, and animal dander, among others.

Gastrointestinal Distress. Any number of allergies can cause stomach upsets, excess gas, constipation, diarrhea, or another gastrointestinal problem. Food allergies are most likely to cause such symptoms, but whenever histamine or some other mediator is released into the body, it can affect the digestive system as well.

Lethargy, Irritability, Depression, and Other Mood Disturbances. More and more attention is being paid, even among mainstream medical doctors, to the relationship between allergies and mood disorders. We now have an understanding of the way that sugar, in particular, affects the way we feel: the sugar "rush" of energy and euphoria is well documented. But now it appears that any substance has the potential to cause an allergy or other hypersensitivity reaction leading to mood swings and disturbances.

Although mainstream doctors are likely to dismiss mood disturbances as part of the allergic syndrome, it is important for you to be aware that what you eat, or fail to eat, as well as what you breathe in or touch, may be affecting your spirit and sense of self. Fortunately, if you choose to explore one or more of the alternatives discussed in this book, it is likely that your whole self—body and mind—will benefit.

Mainstream Diagnosis

Now that you've read about what happens inside your body during an allergic response and about some of the reasons that you might have allergies, we can move on to how modern Western medicine goes about diagnosing and treating your symptoms.

More than likely, you've already visited a doctor—or two or three—in hopes of finding some relief. Perhaps the solutions offered to you have been unsatisfactory, and you still feel unwell even after receiving treatment, or the medication you take for your allergies causes too many unwanted side effects. In the chapters that follow, we explore several more natural and holistic approaches to allergies.

In the meantime, however, it should be noted that if you haven't yet visited a mainstream doctor for an evaluation of your symptoms, you should make an appointment to do so as soon as possible. Without alarming you unduly, there are some serious medical problems that may induce allergylike symptoms, including viral and bacterial infections and certain cancers. Ruling out these conditions, as well as pinpointing as accurately as possible what allergens affect you and how, is among the reasons you should see your physician if you experience allergy symptoms and have not received an official diagnosis.

If you're like most people, your primary care physician will be the first to consider your symptoms. Depending on the severity of the disease and/or the level of her expertise, she may then refer you to an immunologist, a specialist fully trained in general internal medicine who has studied diseases like allergy for an additional two or three years. Other doctors you might visit for treatment include a dermatologist (for skin-related allergies like dermatitis or eczema), a rheumatologist (for related systemic problems such as arthritis), and/or an ear-nose-throat specialist, known as an otorhinolaryngologist (for rhinitis, asthma, or other respiratory symptoms).

Immunology, dermatology, rheumatology, otorhinolaryngology— the list of specialities involved in the treatment of allergies is quite extensive. In fact, this highlights a crucial aspect of disease as viewed by mainstream Western medicine. According to this perspective, each part of the body is considered a distinct and separate entity, largely unconnected to the others. Alternative medicine, on the other hand, views the body as an integrated whole: to distinguish between a problem that causes a skin rash and a problem that causes joint pain—simply because they involve two different areas of the body—is considered an arbitrary and meaningless procedure within these traditions. Perhaps more fundamentally, alternative medicine does not make a sharp distinction between the physical and emotional. Indeed, an alternative medical practitioner is likely to view the state of your mental and emotional health as equal in importance to the state of your physical being.

Despite what might be considered shortcomings in the mainstream approach to a chronic condition like allergy, modern medicine does offer the best technological tools for making a diagnosis—at least from a purely mechanical perspective. When you visit your doctor for an evaluation, you will probably be taken through an exam consisting of some or all of the following:

Medical History. The first step in almost every medical exam, mainstream or alternative, consists of questions asked by the physician or practitioner about your current medical condition, your past experiences, and your family history of disease. He will also delve into aspects of your lifestyle—what kind of work you do (especially in relation to potential allergens in your work environment), your hobbies, the amount of stress under which you live, and what kind of diet you consume on a regular basis, among other issues.

After you and your doctor sort through these issues and discuss aspects of your past medical history (including treatment of previous illnesses unrelated to allergy), your doctor may decide to perform one or more of the following allergy tests:

Skin Tests. The most common test for IgE allergies is the skin test, for which there are several methods. In one test, the doctor places a small amount of the suspected allergen on the skin of either the forearm or the upper arm and then pricks or scratches the area to introduce the allergen beneath the skin surface. Another method involves injecting a tiny amount of an allergen directly into the skin. Results are checked within 15 to 20 minutes. If there is swelling or redness, the test is considered to be positive for that allergen. It should be noted, however, that skin tests are far from foolproof. You may test positive for an allergen, yet have no reaction to that substance in everyday life. The converse is just as likely: you may have no reaction to the skin test, but be highly sensitive to the allergen outside the doctor's office. Generally speaking, skin tests are best used to detect airborne, inhalant allergies and not very useful for food allergies.

RAST. The radioallergosorbent test measures the amount of specific Ig antibodies in your blood. A blood sample is sent to a laboratory where it is exposed to radioactively tagged allergens. A radiation detection device is then used to detect whether the blood has antibodies to the allergen. RAST testing for IgG antibodies is useful in detecting food allergies.

Other Tests. Because increasing numbers of allergists—both mainstream and alternative—recognize that allergies and allergy symptoms are often subtle and difficult to detect, new tests have been developed. In one such test, a food extract is injected under the skin. Instead of looking for an allergic skin reaction, the practitioner looks for such symptoms as discomfort, irritability, drowsiness, or fever.

Perhaps the most reliable and inexpensive way to discover if you are allergic to a substance is to eliminate that substance from your life and see if your symptoms disappear. Of course, if you are allergic to several different foods or chemicals, or if you do not suspect what substance is making you feel unwell, that can be an enormous and perhaps impossible task. Nevertheless, many doctors, both mainstream and alternative, end up relying on just such a strategy to narrow down the type of allergens to which you are sensitive.

Once your doctor narrows down your problem, he or she can suggest a few treatment methods. Unfortunately, scientists have yet to discover a way to realign and rebalance the system of the body most in need of repair: the immune system. Instead, most medicines for allergies focus on alleviating symptoms, often at the expense of general feelings of health and well-being.

Treating Allergies

Throughout this book, you'll find a variety of helpful tips to help you avoid the allergens in your life. It's important, for example, to keep your air-conditioning systems as clean as possible if you want to avoid recirculating offending substances through your home or office. Indeed, avoidance is the most natural method of allergy treatment, and the more allergen-free you can make your environment, the better—both mainstream doctors and alternative medicine practitioners will give you that advice.

In the meantime, it's likely that you've been prescribed one or more of the following medications to help alleviate your symptoms.

Although there appears to be no harm in using these drugs occasionally on a short-term basis, each has its own set of side effects of which
you should be aware.

Antihistamines and Decongestants. For those who suffer
from allergy-related respiratory symptoms, the first treatment usually
involves antihistamines, which reduce the action of histamine in the
body, and decongestants, which reduce the swelling and stuffiness of
nasal passages. Both of these medication types may have unpleasant
side effects, however. Antihistamines frequently cause drowsiness and
dizziness, while decongestants often result in nervousness and nausea.
If taken over a long period of time, decongestants may have a rebound
effect, increasing symptoms rather than decreasing them. Decongestants, since they constrict blood vessels, should be avoided by people
with high blood pressure and vascular disease.

Corticosteroids. These powerful anti-inflammatory drugs come
in various forms, including injection, pill, nasal spray, and cream.
Available mostly by prescription, these drugs can be useful in the treatment of allergy symptoms, but have serious side effects. Muscle weakness, thinning of the skin, high blood pressure, and weight gain are
just a few of the common side effects of long-term corticosteroid use.

Cromolyn Sodium. A noncorticosteroid drug prescribed main-
ly for respiratory allergies, this drug is available in oral form, as a
nasal spray, as eye drops, and in a lung inhaler. Doctors often prescribe
it in advance of the allergy season because the drug must be used for
several weeks before its benefits become apparent. It works by coating the mast cells, thereby preventing the IgE on their surface from
working to release histamine.

Immunotherapy. This type of therapy attempts to desensitize
the system; a series of injections containing the allergen are given over
a period of several months. In theory, you will become less allergic to
the offending substance as time goes on and your body adjusts to it.
However, the process is a long and expensive one, and one that fails
to solve the problem in more than 30 percent of all cases.

As you can see, safe, effective treatment options for allergies are few and far between. In the next chapter, you'll see how other schools of medicine, including those that developed in China and India, view the allergic disease process and treatment.

"No illness which can be treated by diet should be treated by any other means."

Moses Maimonides

3

Choosing an Alternative

$\mathcal{A}$cupuncture. Herbal medicine. Homeopathy. Bodywork. Just a decade ago, such alternatives to mainstream diagnostic and therapeutic techniques formed a relatively small niche in the American health care market. Most of the American general public—to say nothing of medical professionals—appeared either unaware or uninterested in exploring these less "high-tech" methods of treating illness.

As mentioned in Chapter 1, a breakthrough occurred in 1992, when the National Institutes of Health, the United States government's main medical research facility, established its Office of Alternative Medicine. The NIH's decision to put resources into examining the merits of holistic healing techniques was no doubt influenced by reports that Americans were beginning to experiment with alternative medicine in increasing numbers. In fact, in 1995 alone, well over one third of all Americans used some form of alternative medicine as part of their overall health care strategy. As a result, the NIH, private agencies, and medical schools are all now attempting to "catch the wave." More than 20 medical schools now offer some course on holistic and alternative medicine for their students.

Among those who will benefit most from the increased understanding of the principles of alternative medicine are the millions of men, women, and children who suffer from allergies. Alternative medicine, with its emphasis on restoring balance and harmony, offers a host of natural options for you to try. At the same time that you search for a way to alleviate your allergic symptoms, these options also provide you with opportunities to explore different philosophies about the true meaning of health. Instead of settling for merely masking the symptoms of allergies, you may be able to help return your body to a state of equilibrium and balance.

However, you should be aware that in choosing to treat your allergies naturally you'll need to make a larger commitment of time and energy to your health than you may have made in the past. In addition, you may find certain aspects of alternative health to be unfamiliar and, at least at first, perhaps a little uncomfortable. Most forms of alternative therapy, for instance, require that you gain a more intimate knowledge of your body through exercise and massage. You may have to get used to a practitioner examining your body in a different way than your physician has in the past.

In order to gain the most benefit from natural medicine, you'll also need to learn to truly relax your body and mind. For many people, this experience involves exploring emotional and spiritual issues that may have been ignored or suppressed for many years. Although exciting, and ultimately liberating, such work requires some extra motivation and, often, guidance from a trained professional.

If you're like most people who choose to replace or supplement their mainstream health care with more natural approaches, the benefits you'll reap will be well worth the physical and emotional effort you invest. Because of the inherent challenges involved, however, it is important for you to gain some general understanding of the various alternative therapies before you delve into them too deeply. The following quiz will help you sort out some of the questions you may have about alternative medicine and how it might fit into your life.

Your Alternative Medicine Quiz

The questions in this quiz focus on four different categories you should consider when looking for an alternative approach to both treatment of your allergies and your general health. The questions in Part A concern the *physical* aspects of health care; Part B looks at *diet and nutrition;* Part C helps you to focus on your *emotional* and spiritual side; and Part D examines *practical* matters such as finances and access to alternative health care resources.

Answer yes or no to these 16 questions, then check the answer guide that follows to find out what you should look for, or look to avoid, in choosing an alternative therapy.

Part A

1a. I enjoy being massaged and touched by a qualified practitioner. ____
2a. I am willing to experience some discomfort during my treatment. ____
3a. I tolerate needles well. ____
4a. I enjoy physical exercise or am willing to make exercise a part of my future. ____

Part B

1b. I am willing to change my diet. ____
2b. I am willing to learn more about nutrition. ____
3b. I prepare most of my meals at home. ____
4b. I accept that vitamins and minerals are helpful in treating disease. ____

Part C

1c. I accept that emotions play a role in health and healing. ____
2c. I am willing to explore my feelings. ____

3c. I understand that restoring my body to health will
    take time and effort. ____
4c. I now include meditation in my daily life or would like
    to in the future. ____

Part D

1d. I have easy access to one or more alternative practi
    tioners. ____
2d. I have the time and the desire to make and keep a
    schedule of appointments. ____
3d. I have some discretionary income to pay for
    alternative treatments. ____
4d. I can accept treatments that have not been scientifi
    cally proven. ____

THE ANSWER GUIDE

Take a look at your answers. Could you answer "yes" to most of the
questions? Was there one category in which you answered several questions with a "no"? As you'll see in the following guide, your answers to
these questions will help you find the type or types of natural therapy
that best suit your own distinct personality and personal needs.

A. The Physical. Many natural approaches to health care will
require you to establish a new relationship with your body and, in
some cases, with your physician or practitioner. If you dislike being
touched by your doctor, then therapies that concentrate on massage
or other types of physical manipulation may not be for you. Unless
you think you can learn to overcome this aversion, it might be best for
you to avoid Chinese medicine, Ayurvedic medicine, bodywork and
massage, and chiropractic—all of which use physical therapy to a
great extent. Likewise, if you are afraid of needles, then acupuncture
may not appeal to you, unless you can easily put aside your fears.
Being tense and uncomfortable will work directly against the state of
balance and relaxation that is the goal of natural medicine.

However, if one or more of these therapies interest you, you may
want to work through some of your fears and aversions with an
understanding practitioner. She may also be able to help you use the

philosophy behind the treatment without forcing you to undergo any form of therapy that makes you feel uncomfortable.

Finally, you really should be able to answer Question #4 with a yes, whether or not you suffer from allergies. Exercise must become a part of your life if you intend to stay active and healthy for the rest of your life. Depending upon the severity of your allergies and their symptoms, you may have decided that exercise is too taxing, tiring, or disease-inducing to continue. In the end, however, you forsake physical exercise for constant rest only at great risk; you're likely only to become lethargic and despondent—more ill in fact than you feel during your allergy episodes.

B. The Nutritional. As we'll discuss in depth in Chapter 4, the issue of food and allergies is both controversial and crucial, and one with many levels to consider. First, there are food allergies themselves. The body may consider the foods you eat as harmful invaders, thus stimulating the immune system to overreact. Second, certain disturbances or irregularities of the gastrointestinal tract can contribute to the development of a whole host of allergic reactions, by disrupting the internal balance we normally attain with the nutrition we consume. Third, having even the mildest of food allergies can undermine the health of the immune system as a whole, setting the stage for a host of other types of allergies, including exercise-induced asthma, eczema, and chronic headaches. Finally, staying fit and healthy by reducing fat, adding fiber, eliminating (or limiting) sugar and caffeine are just some of the dietary modifications you may need to make in order to bring your body into balance. It will be up to you and your health practitioner to work out the nutritional issues that apply to you.

C. The Emotional. Perhaps the most essential difference between mainstream and alternative medicine is the way these philosophies consider the emotional part of life and health. To understand and then to treat your particular case of allergy, for instance, a holistic practitioner may ask you questions about your sense of self-esteem, your family and professional relationships, and your ability to cope with the stresses in your life. Alternative practitioners consider these issues as important to making an accurate diagnosis and creating an effective treatment plan as any physical symptoms. Because emotional balance is an essential goal of natural medicine, it will help you better cope with your allergies if you can learn to alleviate the stress in your life. To do so, however, will require you to invest time and energy in an area of your life you may well have neglected in the past.

D. The Practical. In addition to the personal factors that may lead you toward a particular form of alternative health care, there are practical matters you should consider as well. First and foremost is how much access you have to alternative resources. If you have to drive several hours to visit a homeopath or acupuncturist, for instance, treating a chronic condition like allergy with these methods might not be possible. Time is another consideration. Many holistic therapies require more frequent visits to a practitioner than you may be used to. Acupuncture and chiropractic are particularly time-consuming, as they usually necessitate continued, frequent appointments, especially at the beginning of therapy. Money is another obstacle for some people, since most forms of health insurance do not cover alternative medicine at this time.

Finally, another practical matter for you to consider is your own commitment to the process of natural healing. Many alternative therapies, despite having been practiced in other cultures for centuries, have not been proven according to certain Western medical standards. (At the same time, however, even many Western drugs have not been really "proven"—anyone who's taken an aspirin for a headache can attest to the fact that sometimes it works, sometimes it doesn't.) If you are someone who needs to understand the scientific basis for a therapy before beginning it, many of these alternatives may not appeal to you at this time. Homeopathy, for instance, is based on an understanding of health and the healing process very different from that provided by the standard medical model. If you choose homeopathic treatment for your allergies, you must be willing to accept the results without fully understanding the process.

As you can see, choosing the type of alternative medicine that is best for you may involve thinking about your life, your body, and your spirit in new ways. The good news is that because natural remedies are safe and relatively free of side effects, you should feel a certain freedom to experiment with different therapies before choosing one over another. You may also decide to mix and match one or more types of approaches instead of using just one alternative method. You may decide to try acupuncture in an effort to restore immune system function over the long term, for example, while at the same time using homeopathic remedies for ongoing symptoms. Fortunately, many holistic practitioners are either specialists in more than one field or are involved in group practices.

No matter what type or types of natural therapy you choose, however, it is essential that you find qualified professionals to treat you. The following section offers a step-by-step guide to locating a reputable practitioner and establishing an effective supportive relationship with him.

Becoming a Wise Alternative Health Care Consumer

Successful treatment of allergies, whether by alternative or mainstream means, requires a partnership between you and the people who treat you, one that is built on mutual trust and respect. You must feel confident in the practitioner's ability to treat your health problems, and she must have vital, accurate information about your medical status and lifestyle in order to provide you with that help. Here are some guidelines to help you become a wise alternative health care consumer.

Obtain an accurate diagnosis. Before you decide upon an alternative therapy or practitioner, you may require certain tests and procedures (see Chapter 2 for more information). These tests are probably best performed by either your family practitioner or an allergy specialist. Bring the results of these tests with you to your first appointment with an alternative practitioner.

Learn as much as possible about the alternative therapy or therapies that appeal to you. Knowledge is power, especially when it comes to health care. Read articles and books about the type of alternative care that appeals to you, talk to friends and acquaintances who use that method, and ask your mainstream physician for his or her opinion.

Check credentials carefully. Unlike those required for mainstream physicians, there are no national licensing requirements for most alternative medicine practitioners at this time. Instead, certification and licensing are done on a state by state basis. Ask your local department of health for the licensing requirements, certification, degrees, and diplomas suggested for a holistic practitioner. For more information about a specific treatment or a specific practitioner, you may call a national association in the specialty field you are considering. (See *Natural Resources*, page 174.)

Interview your prospective practitioner. It is often a good idea to make a short "interview" appointment with a practitioner, even before you decide to be examined by her. During this visit, you should take note of the office itself: Is it clean? Do you feel comfortable there? What are the billing procedures, and is the practitioner willing to set up a payment plan for you? Is the staff friendly and accommodating? Do patient boundaries and confidentiality seem to be respected?

When you meet with the practitioner, ask about how much experience she has had in treating allergies. Find out how accessible she is in between appointments and in case of emergencies. Although it is doubtful that you'll feel completely at ease with the practitioner during this first short meeting, you should be able to tell whether there is potential for a close working relationship. Trust your instincts. If you feel uneasy for any reason, do not feel obligated to continue meeting with her.

Prepare for a long first appointment. Depending on the type of alternative therapy you've chosen to explore, your first appointment (after the prospective interview) may last from 45 to 90 minutes. You'll probably be asked detailed questions about your diet, your medical history, your exercise habits, and your feelings about the work you do and your personal life. Such information is crucial for the practitioner to have before she can develop a treatment plan for you.

At the same time, you should feel comfortable asking your own questions—about your condition, about the procedures the practitioner intends to perform, and even about the questions she is asking of you. Your practitioner should answer these questions in an open and honest way. If you feel you are not being listened to or respected, you have reason to look for another person to treat you.

Get a clear idea of what the suggested course of treatment involves. Discuss what to expect from treatment *before* you agree to it. Ask the practitioner about what to expect in terms of side effects or adverse reactions. Find out how many appointments and how much time it will take before you see symptoms alleviated. Ask how much the treatment will cost and if your insurance is likely to cover it. Although the course of treatment may change as therapy continues, a qualified practitioner should be able to give you a reasonable prognosis, timetable, and cost estimate.

Establish a relationship between your mainstream and alternative practitioners. Ask your mainstream doctor if he would be willing to collaborate with an alternative practitioner on your care—and ask the same thing of any natural therapist you choose. With a chronic, and fairly unpredictable, condition like allergies, it is sensible to have access to the best of both worlds: the life-saving technology and pharmacology of Western medicine in cases of emergency (such as anaphylaxis or severe asthma attacks) and the more subtle, mind/body methods of healing implicit in alternative medicine. In Chapter 13 you'll see how mainstream and alternative medicine can work together to bring you closer to true health—and to freedom from your allergy symptoms.

Don't be afraid to experiment. What works for one person may not work for another, and that is especially true when it comes to health care. If the type of therapy you've chosen does not suit you for any reason, feel free to explore another until you find one or more methods of health care and self-healing that work for you.

Now that you've received a primer of sorts on the basics of alternative medicine, it's time to explore the various techniques used to treat allergies. In the next chapter, you'll find information about food allergies: the symptoms they cause and some of the ways to avoid them.

"Good health
will follow us, if
we follow the
Natural Laws."

J. R. Worsley

Understanding
Food Allergies and
Dietary Influences

4

$\mathcal{M}$ichelle found that when she ate certain foods, allergic symptoms would emerge, including aching in the joints, sinus congestion, and a feeling of "spaciness" or disorientation. An allergist once attempted to treat Michelle; after giving her a skin test, he told her that she was allergic to dust, pollen, and ragweed. However, he insisted that the skin tests did not show that she had allergies to wheat, corn, tomatoes, dairy, or yeast, all of which brought on symptoms regularly. He offered her antihistamines and sent her home.

Frustrated and losing too much weight because of self-imposed restrictions in her diet, Michelle saw a doctor who practiced nutritional medicine. The first thing this doctor did was to confirm that people could indeed have reactions to foods that will not show up on standard skin allergy testing. He then performed a blood test called an IgG RAST that showed different immune reactions than the skin testing, which showed only IgE response. He explained that although the RAST test was not perfect, it would serve as a good guide to the foods that might cause Michelle problems. He also asked her to keep a careful "diet diary"—a record of every morsel of food she consumed and what symptoms (if any) it caused.

When the tests came back, it turned out that wheat, rye, and other grains, as well as corn, tomatoes, green beans, peanuts, and yeast caused allergic responses in Michelle. To double-check the test results, the doctor had Michelle withdraw all the offending foods for three weeks. For the first time in years, Michelle felt she could breathe easily, think clearly, and exercise regularly without upsetting her system.

As she added the foods back into her diet, she felt her symptoms return. The doctor explained that certain blood and stool tests showed her to have yeast in her system, which kept her immune system over-stimulated. Past treatment with antibiotics for skin problems and sinus infections contributed to the yeast problem.

To counteract the yeast in Michelle's system, the doctor prescribed certain supplements, including an extract of grapefruit seed, concentrated garlic capsules, and intestinal bacteria called acidophilus. He asked her not to consume any sugar, any foods with yeast in them, or any fermented substance, such as alcohol, vinegar, or malt. He also gave her digestive enzymes (to assist her digestion) and several other nutritional supplements to improve her immune system function. Finally, he provided Michelle with a rotation diet that allowed her to eat all of her problem foods (except for yeast)—as long as she didn't eat them any more often than every fourth day.

During the next several months, Michelle found her symptoms had declined and her overall health improved. She also found she could tolerate foods that she once had to avoid altogether. For the next year, she continued to take her supplements, avoided yeasted foods, and never ate any food two days (rather than four) in a row. Because she felt so much better, these small sacrifices seemed a small price to pay for her increased vitality.

ALLERGY TIP

Try to make exercise a regular part of your life. Not only does exercise reduce stress, but it also helps to relieve allergy symptoms by helping the body get rid of excess water and toxins. Choose an activity that you enjoy so that you'll be more likely to stick with the program.

Michelle is one of millions of Americans who find that certain foods, or combinations of foods, cause their immune system to over-react, leaving them feeling ill and uncomfortable. Because food allergies produce such a wide variety of symptoms—some of them quite subtle—and are caused by such a wide variety of substances, they remain the subject of some controversy among doctors, patients, and even alternative practitioners.

Food allergy symptoms can occur throughout the body and range from a mild stomachache to sudden death. If the allergy reaction occurs when the food moves into the stomach and intestines, the symptoms can include nausea, vomiting, bowel cramps, and diarrhea. The reaction can occur in the respiratory system, causing asthma attacks and breathing problems. Skin symptoms, including hives, itching, and swelling, also may result from eating a food your body recognizes as an enemy. Headaches, irritability, hyperactivity, and mood swings have all been linked to food allergy.

Any kind of food—fruits and vegetables, meats and fish, nuts, grains, sugar, caffeine, alcohol, dairy products, and additives and preservatives—can cause an allergic reaction by directly triggering an immune response or by more subtly undermining the immune system's ability to function properly. In fact, allergists are discovering that your body can respond in several different ways to foods it perceives as foreign and dangerous.

Fixed Reaction. In this case, your body responds in a relatively stable and similar way to each exposure to a food allergen. Fifteen minutes after eating a strawberry, you break out in hives, for instance, or an hour after eating Chinese food made with the additive MSG, you develop a splitting headache. With fixed reactions, you are more likely to know to which foods you are allergic and what type of reaction to expect.

Cumulative Reaction. A cumulative reaction occurs after you've been exposed to a relatively large quantity of a particular substance, usually over a long period of time. For instance, if your immune system is sensitive to gluten (a substance found in bread products), you may develop a severe allergy if you eat lots of bread and pasta every day. In fact, the most commonly ingested foods—wheat, dairy, and yeast—also trigger the most food allergies. If you eat a wide variety of foods and consume only limited amounts of gluten on an occasional basis, your immune system may be able to "ignore" the disturbance and digest the food without incident. Also, one specific food allergen by itself may not cause a reaction, but when combined with other substances or environmental factors will trigger a more pronounced response. It is possible for other allergens—such as pollen or pet dander—to disrupt the immune system and leave you more vulnerable to food allergies, and vice versa.

Variable Reaction. As you may have experienced yourself, allergic reactions are not always predictable. One day, you can have a salad chock full of tomatoes and enjoy it; then the next, you'll have just a slice of tomato and break out in terrible itchy hives. Factors such as your state of mind and your level of stress may affect your reactions to food. The environment, including the presence of toxic substances like cigarette smoke or other pollutants, may also cause you to be more sensitive to food allergens.

Anaphylaxis. This often fatal reaction to an allergen most often occurs in people allergic to nuts or shellfish, which appear to be among the most potent food allergens. Generally speaking, anaphylaxis is not the first reaction someone has to an allergen; instead, a buildup of antibodies against the substance must occur before you would experience this violent response.

Food Addiction. If you find yourself in an uncontrollable cycle of craving a particular food, then ingesting it and experiencing unpleasant physical reactions that, upon subsiding, are only replaced by more craving, it is possible that you are, in fact, allergic to that food.

Food Allergies: The Difficulty of Diagnosis

Although it is becoming increasingly clear that what we eat has widespread effects on our day-to-day health, diagnosing a food allergy is a difficult process for even the most attuned and experienced practitioners. The challenges are fourfold:

First, even those of us who consume relatively regular and limited diets eat a number of different foods, or at least foods that contain a wide variety of substances. Processed foods—any foods that are not in their natural, raw states when you buy them—contain any number of ingredients that you might not expect, as well as a host of preservatives and additives. A look at the label on a package of "all natural" macaroni and cheese, for example, will show you how many ingredients it takes to make this product: elbow style pasta (made with whole wheat flour), corn flour, Cheddar cheese (pasteurized milk, cheese cultures, salt, and enzymes), sweet whey, buttermilk, annatto extract, and natural flavor. Any one of these substances could trigger an allergic reaction in a susceptible individual; so could the food colorings, preservatives, artificial sweeteners, and other ingredients found in so many of the most common food products around today.

Second, many foods cause adverse reactions that are not technically allergies. Some people, for instance, become nauseous and bloated after drinking milk. What they suffer from is lactose intolerance—an inability to digest milk sugar—rather than an allergy to milk. Food poisoning caused by spoilage or contamination can be also confused with an allergic reaction. Differentiating between sensitivities, allergies, and other reactions can be quite a challenge for both doctors and those people who suffer from them.

Third, symptoms of food allergies can be very subtle and diverse, and match those of other conditions. You may not realize that an allergy to wheat or chocolate causes your periodic headaches, for example, or that you become irritable after foods containing certain food additives or contaminants. This is especially true if your reactions are more emotional than physical. You're much more likely to attribute your sudden irritability to something your boss said to you than to the food you ate at lunch.

Finally, even a slight immune sensitivity to a food you eat often may disrupt your whole body, so much so that you develop a host of allergies to any number of nonfood substances. Therefore, you're more likely to be treated for hay fever rather than the underlying problem of an allergy to gluten.

In fact, when doctors diagnose a food allergy, they usually start by looking for other signs of allergy-related disease, such as a family history or an existing allergy such as hay fever. The doctor or practitioner will also look for symptoms that occur repeatedly after you eat a given food. If a suspected food is identified, the doctor may use the tests described in Chapter 2, primarily skin testing and RAST, for more information.

Perhaps the most useful test for food allergy is called the *elimination challenge diet*, in which the suspected food is first banned and then put back into the diet to see whether symptoms occur. To help decide which food or foods should be eliminated from the diet, you may be asked to keep a detailed food diary for a week or two before you start the challenge. In this diary, you would keep track of every single substance you put in your mouth (including the foods you eat, the liquids you imbibe, and any antacids or other medications you take), the time of day you consume it, your state of mind or activity at the time you eat it, and any mood changes or physical symptoms you feel during the day.

Michelle kept a diary for about two weeks at the beginning of her treatment with the nutritionist. A typical day's entry looked like this one:

Monday's Food Diary

8:00 A.M.   *Breakfast*: Doughnut, coffee (reading morning paper, feeling calm)

10:00 A.M.   Feeling jittery and a little spacey

12:30 P.M.   *Lunch*: Tuna sandwich with lettuce and tomato on whole-wheat toast, milk (working on report for business meeting, feeling stressed and anxious)

2:00 P.M.   Feeling tired and achy

3:00 P.M.   *Snack*: Coffee, corn muffin (craving a pick-me-up, still feeling a little anxious)

4:30 P.M.   Feeling less tired, but still a little achy in joints

7:00 P.M.   *Dinner:* Fish and brown rice stir-fry, glass of wine (finally relaxed)

8:30 P.M.   Getting sleepy but feeling better

When Michelle's nutritionist took a look at Michelle's entire diary, he saw that Michelle reacted quite strongly to certain foods, primarily wheat, corn, and tomatoes, just as she had thought. The nutritionist suspected, however, that Michelle's problems were exacerbated by how much and how often she ate the offending substances: breakfast, lunch, and her afternoon snack all contained wheat and yeasted products. As we'll discuss a little later in the chapter, when Michelle learned to vary her diet and space out her consumption of certain substances, she was able to eat her favorite foods on an occasional basis while maintaining her health.

If you feel you might have an allergy to one or more foods, you should begin to keep a food diary—even before you visit a nutritionist or other health professional. That way, you'll come to your first appointment armed with very specific and helpful information that will help your health practitioner choose appropriate further testing, such as skin tests and RASTs.

Once you and your doctor identify the food or foods that may be causing your problems, you will probably begin the elimination diet challenge. On an elimination diet, you will exclude a given food or foods from your diet for seven to eight days or until your symptoms have improved for at least two days. Then, you reintroduce each food in pure form, one food at a time, and note your symptoms. If you feel worse when a food is returned to your diet, the food becomes suspected of—if not confirmed as—being an allergen. You'll withhold that food and wait 24 to 48 hours until you feel better, then try consuming another eliminated food to see how you react to that substance.

As you embark upon this test, keep in mind the following tips:

Read all labels carefully. As we'll discuss a little later, we should all strive to eat as much fresh food, uncorrupted by preservatives or additives, as possible. But that is a task that gets harder and harder to achieve every day. Thus it is necessary for you to look carefully at food labels, noting all ingredients and their amounts, when you keep your food diary and when you undertake the elimination diet.

Plan your menus and shop in advance. To avoid eating an eliminated food by accident or on the run, make sure you have everything you need to eat well for at least a week. If you spend lots of time out of the house, be sure to bring "safe" snacks along with you in case you get hungry. If at all possible, avoid restaurant eating altogether for the week; you never can be sure what ingredients are used that might sabotage your attempt to accurately identify potential allergens.

Keep track of everything you consume. Toothpaste (if you swallow it), mouthwash, medications (both over-the-counter and prescription), and chewing gum all contain ingredients to which you

---

ALLERGY TIP

When planning a healthy diet, try to vary your menu as much as possible. Not only is it the best way to ensure adequate nutrition, but you're also less likely to overload your body with any one substance and will thus reduce your chances of having an allergic reaction to that food.

might be sensitive. If one of the foods you are avoiding is sugar, for instance, you should avoid taking antacids, which frequently contain sugar, or swallowing mouthwash, for the same reason.

Once you've identified and confirmed the foods that disturb your system, you have a few options in terms of treating your allergies. We discuss those options next.

Treatment for Food Allergies

In the next several chapters, you'll learn about a variety of alternative treatments for all types of allergies, food allergies included. In the meantime, here are two suggestions for lowering your chances of experiencing an allergic reaction triggered by the foods you eat:

Avoidance. The simplest way to avoid triggering an allergic response to a particular food is to eliminate it entirely from your diet. In some cases, such a strategy is easy to accomplish: if you are allergic to only strawberries, for instance, you simply don't ever have to eat another berry in your life. However, an allergy to wheat can rule out a whole range of products—both obvious ones such as breads and cakes and less obvious ones like hot dogs, canned soups, and noodles, which often have wheat as an ingredient. An allergy to nuts or to meat such as beef may rule out equally long lists of related food. Organizations such as the National Academy of Allergy and Immunology and the American Allergy Association have prepared lists of foods to be avoided when a specific food allergy is diagnosed. They also have listings of companies that manufacture prepared foods for restricted diets and offer cookbooks with recipes that do not require such ingredients as milk, eggs, or wheat. See *Natural Resources*, page 174, for more information.

Rotation Diet. If you truly feel you cannot live without eating another strawberry at some point in your life, or if you have multiple food allergies to common substances, you may find that a rotation diet is most helpful. A rotation diet systematically varies the food you eat as much as possible, thereby reducing both the amount and the frequency with which you consume foods your immune system recognizes as allergens.

The number of days between eating foods to which you might have a sensitivity or allergy depends on a number of factors. Some doctors recommend not eating any one food (whether or not it is an allergen) more often than every two to four days. We recommend that you visit a nutritionist who specializes in food allergies to help you sort through a strategy that will work for you

In addition to following one or both of these prescriptions directly related to your food allergy, it is also important for you to take the time to look at your eating habits in general. "You are what you eat" may have become a cliche, but it is one with special meaning in late twentieth-century America.

Eating for Fitness and Health

Why are we Americans so plagued with bad eating habits? Although most of us tend to blame our own lack of willpower, we can look to a number of outside influences that conspire to turn us into a nation of unhealthy eaters. Perhaps the most obvious and pervasive one is the television set. Not only does it entice us into spending too many hours sitting in a heap in front of it, but it constantly sells us apparently delicious, time-saving delectables—most of which are laden with fat and empty calories. The fact that our lives tend to be hectic and disjointed, leaving us with little time to plan our meals and enjoy them together with friends and family, also contributes to our increasingly poor eating habits and large waistlines.

At the same time, we read headlines every day about the dangers of food—sugar is bad, fat is worse, margarine is better than butter (one day), then a health risk (the next). The mixed messages we receive tend to either confuse us to the point that we no longer even try to learn about nutrition or turn us into hypervigilant, slightly paranoid "food avoiders." In all this, we forget that food is good for us; it's meant to be enjoyed and savored at every meal.

Food is nourishment. The nutrients in the food you eat are the catalysts for millions of major and minor miracles—the beating of your heart, the birth of an idea, the appreciation of taste and smell—that take place within the chemistry lab that is your body. Food is also a source of pleasure. We do not eat merely to ingest the various nutrients, vitamins, and minerals we need to survive. Instead, eating is a supremely sensual activity: we smell food's aromas, taste its flavors, admire its colors and textures, and feel its consistency inside our mouths. Depending on the circumstances, our sense of hearing is also stimulated by the conversation of our tablemates or the sounds of soothing dinner music.

As you consider your dietary habits, ask yourself these questions: Do you take the time to enjoy the sensual aspects of eating, or do you simply think of food as fuel for the body? Do you eat only those things that taste good without considering their nutritional value? Are there foods that you enjoy eating but which seem to exacerbate your arthritis symptoms or otherwise upset your system? Depending on how you answer these questions, you may discover that your approach to eating could use a little readjustment, especially if those habits have left you eating too much of the wrong kinds of food. The following tips might help you to look at your daily eating habits in new and healthier ways.

MAINTAIN A HEALTHY WEIGHT

Many people with food allergies tend to be underweight (because they attempt to eliminate too many foods in order to alleviate their symptoms) or overweight (because their allergies create a food addiction or because they tend to overindulge in foods to which they are not allergic). If you need to gain or lose weight, talk to your practitioner about creating a calorie-sensible eating plan.

Fortunately, there are some relatively simple techniques that may help you maintain your weight over the long term. Try building one or more of these habits into your life:

Eat five to six small meals a day. The more often you eat, the less hungry you'll be and the less food you'll eat at each meal.

Learn to eat breakfast, a midmorning snack, lunch, an afternoon snack, dinner, and a before-bedtime snack.

Keep portions small. Americans typically eat twice as much food as recommended: one cup of pasta represents *two* servings of bread. Six ounces of fish or meat represents *two* servings of protein. Until you become familiar with proper serving sizes, you might want to weigh and measure your food.

Halve your intake of oils while doubling your intake of fresh vegetables and whole grains. Although we're taking some positive steps in the right direction, fat remains a ubiquitous part of the average American diet. One way fat enters our bodies is through salad dressings and sauces. Instead of drenching your vegetables and grains, place a tablespoonful on the edge of your plate and dab your food with it, bite by bite. Sprinkle vegetables with lemon juice and spices for additional flavor.

Consume all good things in moderation. Unless you have a specific allergy or sensitivity or have a problem with yeast infections, no food should be off-limits for you. Instead of spending precious time, energy, and stress avoiding foods that society considers "bad," you should work on integrating small amounts of those forbidden foods into your diet. An occasional piece of chocolate cake (as long as you're not allergic to any of its ingredients) will do far less damage to your body than the stress you may put yourself under just trying to resist it.

Plan and cook ahead. If you make an effort to organize your eating by creating a menu for the week, shopping, and even cooking ahead of time, it's likely that you'll enjoy your mealtimes more, successfully avoid any possible food triggers, and broaden the variety of foods you eat and enjoy—all at the same time.

Add variety to your diet. By eating lots of different kinds of food during the day, not only will you improve your chances of getting all the nutrients you need and of avoiding overloading on any one allergen, you're also likely to find yourself enjoying your diet more than ever before. At least once a week, try a new food—an exotic fruit or vegetable, for instance—or cook a different dish. Of course, it's important to identify possible allergens before you experiment too much, but generally speaking, the more varied your diet, the better.

Eat foods that leave you feeling healthy and well. In addition to avoiding foods to which you are allergic, it's important to recognize that you may be sensitive in more subtle ways to other kinds—or amounts—of food. Pay attention to how you feel after you eat your meals. If you're often groggy and uncomfortable, you may be eating too much, failing to eat a balanced diet, or consuming food that doesn't agree with your particular body makeup. Nutritious food, prepared well and eaten in a relaxed atmosphere, should nourish your body and your soul.

Be alert to the potential dangers of sugar and yeast. If you have a food allergy or, indeed, any kind of allergy, you should pay special attention to two particular substances found in high quantities in the average American diet: sugar and yeast. As you attempt to reorganize your diet, keep in mind these facts about sugar and yeast:

Sugar: The average American consumes about one-half cup of sugar each day, or more than 100 pounds per year. In addition to our penchant for sweets, sugar has found its way into all sorts of apparently benign foods, like breakfast cereals, soups, catsup, luncheon meats, peanut butter, and salad dressings. Eliminating or dramatically reducing the amount of refined sugar in your diet may be one of the most healthy habits you can develop.

In addition to the fact that sugar contains nutritionally empty, potentially fattening calories, many allergists now believe that sugar addiction may be one of the most common food allergies around. Double-blind studies have shown that many people have allergic reactions to refined cane sugar (the kind found in most foods) and not to sugars made from corn or beets. Furthermore, sugar and other simple carbohydrates tend to feed another substance in the body that can wreak havoc on our immune systems: a substance known as yeast.

Yeast: Yeast (particularly the species known as *Candida albicans*) is a substance that lives in our bodies naturally, primarily in the mouth, esophagus, intestines, vagina, and skin. As long as our immune system keeps it in balance, *Candida* levels stay in check and the substance does no harm to the internal functioning of the body. However, should the immune system become weak for any reason—such as during a fight against a major infection or through immunosuppressive drugs or an immunodeficient disease like AIDS—the yeast can multiply, forming colonies that further challenge the immune system. New research shows that chronic yeast infection may lead someone to develop severe allergies to inhalants (like pollen and ragweed), foods of all kinds, medications, and chemicals. In fact, the person who is sensitive to a wide variety of substances is more likely to have an allergy to yeast, or have a chronic yeast infection, than someone sensitive to just one or two allergens.

Talk to your doctor or practitioner about your potential for having yeast-related allergy problems, especially if you have a history of yeast infections (thrush, vaginal yeast infections, etc.), if you have a long history of taking antibiotics (especially tetracycline) or birth control pills, or if you suffer from an autoimmune disorder such as multiple sclerosis, rheumatoid arthritis, or Crohn's disease. If yeast plays a part in your health problems, your practitioner may suggest the following strategies:

1. Reduce exposure to all yeast foods and their relatives in your diet. This includes baked goods raised with baker's yeast, products enriched with brewer's yeast, vinegars and products containing vinegar, fermented beverages (like alcohol, ginger ale, root beer), foods high in mold content such as aged cheeses and sour cream, and malted products such as cereals, candy, and malted milk drinks.
2. Begin a low-carbohydrate diet. Yeast colonies cannot live and reproduce well on proteins and fats alone; they need carbohydrates to thrive. If you have an allergy to yeast, or if you have a *Candida albicans* infection, try to keep your daily intake of carbohydrates down to about 60–80 grams a day—the equivalent of about one cup of pasta. Your doctor or alternative health practitioner will provide you with special dietary guidelines and instructions to help you create a healthy, low-carb eating plan.

The ABCs of Nutritional Supplements

Although in the best of all possible worlds we would receive all the nutrients we need from the food we eat, many researchers believe that supplementing our diets with certain vitamins and minerals is an important component in any successful treatment of allergies. The following nutrients are those most often mentioned in this connection:

Zinc. Studies in laboratory animals as well as in humans have shown that deficiencies in this trace mineral depress the immune system, leaving the body more vulnerable to both allergies and infections. Zinc, as well as vitamin A (see below), plays an important role in the production of IgA, the gastrointestinal antibody secreted from the salivary glands in the mouth and from cells that line the digestive tract. When IgA binds to an allergen, it keeps it from being absorbed into the bloodstream and thus from causing an allergic reaction. Zinc is also necessary for protein synthesis and carbohydrate digestion. Finally, zinc also protects mucous membrane linings, and it helps convert pre-vitamin A (beta carotene) to vitamin A. The RDA for zinc is about 15 milligrams. (Meat, liver, eggs, and seafoods are the best dietary sources of zinc.)

Vitamin A. Vitamin A also acts to increase the body's production of IgA, thus helping to reduce immune system reactions to food allergens. Vitamin A promotes good vision, helps form and maintain healthy skin and mucous membranes, and may protect against certain cancers. Liver, eggs, carrots, tomatoes, and fish are particularly rich sources of vitamin A.

Flavonoids. The flavonoids are a group of plant pigments largely responsible for the colors of fruits and flowers. In addition, they serve to protect plants against environmental stress and modify the human body's reaction to allergens and infectious agents. Flavonoids also have antiinflammatory properties. Among the most important flavonoids for people with allergies are those responsible for the colors of blueberries, blackberries, cherries, grapes, and other plants. Among their properties is the ability to increase vitamin C levels within cells, decrease the leakiness and breakage of small blood vessels, and protect against free-radical damage.

Antioxidants. Found in rich supply in fruits and vegetables, vitamins and minerals called antioxidants fight against molecules known as free radicals.

Other natural antioxidant substances are found in plants such as pine bark and seeds such as grape pips, both high in a rich antioxidant substance called pycnogenol. Free radicals are unstable molecules created by normal chemical processes in the body (like the immune response to allergies) or environmental influences like radiation and cigarette smoke. In an attempt to stabilize themselves, these unstable molecules try to combine with nonradical molecules in the body. By doing so, they often damage the membranes and internal structures of healthy cells—including immunoglobulins, the B cells that produce them, and other immune system cells.

In the body, the most damaging free radicals are derived from the chemical process by which oxygen is utilized inside the cells. Antioxidants, such as vitamins C and E, beta-carotene (which the body converts to vitamin A), and the mineral selenium, are substances that render these free radicals harmless. The more fresh fruits and vegetables containing these substances you consume, the better off your general health. Even if antioxidants cannot solve your allergy problem, they can help you remain strong so that coping with allergies will be less stressful.

Recommended dosages of vitamin C supplements range from 250 to 3,000 mg per day. Please note, however, vitamin C can be quite acidic; the more you take, the more risk you have for developing stomach irritation. At the same time, keep in mind that aspirin and antihistamines both tend to deplete vitamin C from the body, which is another reason you might want to supplement your daily intake of this vitamin. Recommended dosages of vitamin E supplements range from 200 to 800 IU (international units) per day.

Vitamins B_1, B_3, and B_6 are particularly helpful in reducing anxiety, which can help alleviate the cycle of frustration and discomfort many people with allergies endure. Foods rich in B vitamins include fish, nuts, grains, eggs, liver, and lean meats. If you and your practitioner feel you aren't getting enough B vitamins in your diet, you may want to take about 25–100 mg of vitamin B complex (available in both a one-dose time-release form or several smaller doses throughout the day). If you are particularly anxious or under stress, you can add up to 3,000 mg a day of vitamin B_3 (also known as niacin), as long as you remain under the care of a doctor. Niacin may affect the liver and thus requires close monitoring.

Now that you've read about how to improve your diet by avoiding foods that may be harmful to your health while bolstering your own internal health-promoting faculties, you can now explore another tradition of medicine and healing developed in China.

"The most basic

force underlying

all of nature

is intelligence."

Deepak Chopra

5

Acupuncture and
Chinese Medicine

....

*E*very year, Marta spent four miserable months suffering
from allergies that made her head feel like lead and her nose light up
like a light bulb. Doctors had tested her for all sorts of allergies
when she was a child. Skin testing showed that various pollens,
trees, grasses, dust, and many other substances found inside and
outside caused her immune system to overreact. She took several different types of antihistamines and decongestants, but found that
they made her very jumpy and anxious. Finally, she decided to visit a
practitioner of Chinese medicine.

The doctor asked her many questions about her allergy symptoms, including what brought them on, what time of day or year she
suffered most, whether heat or cold helped or hurt her sinuses. The
practitioner asked her to describe other aspects of her health as well,

such as her digestion, sleep patterns, and menstrual history. He then took Marta's pulse for a long time and examined her tongue.

The Chinese diagnosis focused on what the practitioner called "damp heat." Marta's digestive organs had always given her problems, including gas, bloating, and episodes of diarrhea and spasm. Her internist had told her this condition was "irritable bowel syndrome." According to Chinese medical philosophy, however, this meant that the products of digestion were not being processed but instead accumulated as mucus. In Marta's case, inflammation combined with the mucous congestion in her head, leading to the damp heat diagnosis.

The practitioner prescribed several different treatments for Marta. First, he set up acupuncture sessions designed to lessen the acute inflammation of her sinuses. Acupuncture points targeted included those over the sinuses themselves, which resulted in almost immediate opening of her clogged nose and ears. In addition, points on the legs and feet, which corresponded to the stomach and spleen channel points, drained the dampness and cooled the inflammation. Subsequently, the practitioner used points to tonify or strengthen the digestion, at one point adding moxa—an herb heated over the skin—which further assisted in drying up Marta's damp condition.

In addition to her acupuncture sessions, Marta also took Chinese herbs, including a pill called Pe Min Kan Wan and a powder called Xanthium. Together, they seemed to do at least as well as her decongestant in alleviating symptoms and with fewer side effects. Later, the practitioner added an herbal tincture that had cardamom and other herbs in it.

Marta continued her acupuncture visits through the summer. When fall arrived—normally her worst allergy season—Marta barely noticed it, although she did need to use an antihistamine a few times. In addition to finding relief from her allergies, Marta also noticed that she had less gas and bloating after eating, and her digestion in general felt better.

Like Marta, you may find that acupuncture and Chinese herbal medicine will help to resolve your allergic condition. Later in this chapter, we talk more about how acupuncture works and how to find a qualified practitioner. In the meantime, however, it may interest you to know that acupuncture belongs to a rich and multilayered approach to health and healing, one that encompasses every aspect of your being—mind, soul, and body.

The Philosophy of Chinese Medicine

More than 2,500 years ago, an unknown group of healers compiled a text known as *The Yellow Emperor's Canon of Internal Medicine*. This first major treatise on Chinese medicine that has come down to us outlines an approach to life and health still practiced by more than one quarter of the world's population and now followed by more and more Americans every year. It is a complex, all-encompassing philosophy based on Taoist tenets.

At its heart, the Chinese philosophy of health views humanity, and each individual human, as part of a larger creation—the universe itself. Each of us is subject to the same laws that govern all of nature. In fact, Chinese medicine refers to the flow of bodily fluid and energy as channels and rivers, and the state of the body as a whole in terms of the natural elements.

According to Chinese philosophy, human beings represent the juncture between heaven and earth, and thus a fusion of cosmic and earthly forces. Indeed, human beings *are* nature, and thus subject to its cyclic patterns and ebbs and flows. The state of your health, as well as the health of the universe and the planet, are all connected through the same unified system known as the *Tao*, or "the way." When any part of this unified whole become unbalanced, natural disasters (such as floods or droughts) or human disease may occur. What injures the earth injures each of us, and to heal the body is to foster the health and well-being of the whole universe.

YIN-YANG AND THE FIVE CLIMATES

In Chinese medicine, your ability to maintain a balanced and harmonious internal environment determines the state of your health.

Internal harmony is expressed through the principle of yin-yang, in which two opposing forces have united to create everything in the universe. Yin has connotations of cold, dark, and wet, while yang is warm, bright, and dry. Yin is quiet, static, and inactive while yang is dynamic, active, and expansive. In a human being, parts of the body are ascribed more yin or more yang qualities, as are all physiological processes and diseases, including allergies. Hot, swollen sinuses with thick mucus are considered more yang, for instance, while dry coughing and weakness is more yin.

Furthermore, Chinese medicine compares internal response patterns of the body to external climatic conditions; in other words, according to this philosophy, climate exists internally as well as externally. Cold, for instance, makes things contract. Contracted blood vessels constrict the circulation, leading to a feeling of chill. If you describe having a chill to a practitioner of Chinese medicine, he or she will describe your condition as *cold*, regardless of whether or not actual exposure to cold caused the condition, or whether or not you have the common cold. There are five climates in Chinese medicine: cold, wind, heat, dampness, and dryness. In most cases of allergies, wind is considered to have invaded the channels of the body (called meridians, as described below), causing some of the respiratory and other symptoms.

Connecting and motivating yin and yang and the Five Climates is a flow of energy through our bodies and through the universe, a force known as qi. Keeping a balanced, rich supply of qi coursing through the body is essential to health, according to the traditions and philosophy of Chinese medicine.

QI: THE LIFE FORCE

According to Chinese philosophy, yin-yang imbalance is at the root of all disease. Yin-yang can become disturbed when the flow of energy through the body—the energy known as qi (pronounced "chee")—is interrupted or blocked in some way. As mentioned, in Chinese medicine, qi is the energy essential for life. All of your body's functions are manifestations of qi, and your health is determined by a sufficient, balanced, and unimpeded flow of qi. Qi ensures bodily function by keeping blood

ALLERGY TIP

If you have a food allergy, be sure to call the hosts of any dinner party you're going to attend, well in advance of the event, to alert them to your special needs. If they plan to serve something apt to make you feel ill, offer to bring something you know is safe for you to eat. Above all, don't be so embarrassed or cavalier about your allergies that you risk your health by not taking simple precautions.

and body fluids circulating to warm the body, fight disease, and protect the body against negative forces from the external environment.

Qi circulates through the body along a continuous circuit of pathways known as meridians. These meridians flow along the surface of the body and through the internal organs. When you are healthy, you have an abundance of qi flowing smoothly through the meridians and organs, which allows your body to function in balance and harmony. If qi becomes blocked along one of your meridians, however, the organ or tissue meant to be nourished by this energy will not receive enough qi to perform its functions. By locating where in the body qi is blocked, and by releasing it through acupuncture, acupressure, herbs, and exercises, practitioners of Chinese medicine attempt to restore proper energy flow to the body.

In doing so, practitioners distinguish conditions caused by a deficiency or weakness of qi from those caused by excess qi. In general, allergies result from a weak condition. Either the lung is weak, leading to respiratory symptoms (sneezing, dry coughing, wheezing); the spleen is weak, leading to dampness and mucous accumulation (stuffy nose, digestive problems); or the kidney is weak, leading to a vulnerability and exhaustion of the immune and nervous system, as well as inflammation rising to the head and surface of the body. More often, aspects of all three types of qi weakness are present.

Diagnosis and Treatment of Allergies

Like most other branches of natural medicine, Chinese medicine provides no standard diagnostic signs or treatment plans. Instead, the practitioner will make an evaluation of your condition based on your own unique constitution and energy level. Essentially, doctors of Chinese medicine attempt to treat all symptoms of disease by restoring yin-yang and a healthy qi flow to the body. Since allergies are considered a weak condition, therapy would attempt to bolster or tonify qi in the organs and meridians deficient in qi.

The Five Element Theory as taught by modern Taoist philosopher and acupuncture expert Professor J. R. Worsley adds an interesting perspective about allergies to this discussion. According to Worsley, people allergic to many foods and/or many environmental factors may have a weakness in what is called the "heart protector." The heart protector—an energy field within the body—has the role of guarding our heart physically (in terms of our exposure to the external world), emotionally (in terms of our ability to receive and experience intimacy), and mentally (in terms of our communication with others). When it's functioning well, the heart-protector energy allows us to receive what's appropriate and keep out what's not—whether what is inappropriate is food, environmental substances, or even ideas, lovers, or other people's emotions.

In many people's lives, however, something breached the heart protector when they were quite young. Such a breach might be overt, such as in sexual abuse or incest, or subtle, as occurs in a family structure that does not respect boundaries of privacy. Once the protection is breached, it never functions quite as well, just as a door broken from its hinge can never be repaired 100 percent. Thus the person is never quite able to distinguish what is safe from what might be dangerous. The end result is someone whose system reacts to everyday substances, even such nourishing ones as wheat or corn or the air you breathe, not "knowing" whether or not it is safe. Multiple sensitivities result. Emotionally, such people may become very guarded in their relationships or, conversely, engage in unsafe sexual behavior. Such people might be very sensitive to environmental or emotional factors around them, again showing a hypervigilant state.

In order to focus on your particular problem, the practitioner of Chinese medicine will take a medical history and then perform a complete physical exam. Like most of us used to the more mainstream approach to the medical exam, you might find a visit to a Chinese medical office a bit on the exotic side. You may pick up the slightly sweet smell of burning moxa, the herb frequently used as part of acupuncture treatments. Even after you sit down with the practitioner, you might be surprised by the course the appointment takes. First, you'll probably spend far more time than usual discussing the symptoms that brought you to the visit in the first place. The practitioner will ask you to be very specific about your symptoms, asking you when your allergies tend to come on, what they feel like, and what tends to make them feel better or worse. He or she may ask you more general questions about how you react to heat or cold, dampness and dryness, and seasonal variations; you may be asked about day to night changes in mood and feelings of well-being. Other questions might concern bowel movements, menstruation, and eating and drinking habits. Your answers to these questions will give the doctor an idea of what part of your physiology might be affecting your immune system, leading to allergies.

The physical examination that follows may also be a bit different from what you might be used to. A practitioner of Chinese medicine places a great deal of importance on listening to your pulse. In fact, she will feel 12 different pulses, 6 on each side, and each related to a different organ in the body. The pulses also relate to meridians, the energy pathways through the body, which, if blocked, may result in disease or pain. The practitioner may also spend time looking at your tongue. According to the tenets of Chinese medicine, the tongue's coating, color, and shape reveal much about your body. By examining your tongue, the doctor is also attempting to locate where in your body qi flow has been disrupted. The abdomen also is important in some acupuncture systems, and therefore a Chinese practitioner may press on points in the stomach to feel for tenderness, for warm or cool areas, and for a pulse in the umbilicus (belly button).

If your heart-protector energy is weak, the physical exam will show a tightness across the upper back and tenderness next to the breastbone. You probably tend to have shallow breathing and a coolness to your belly. You may frequently complain of numbness or coldness of your hands and feet. These are all signs of energy wrapped too tightly around the chest to protect the heart and, therefore, energy that is not circulating to other parts of the body.

After performing these exams, as well as observing your demeanor, way of moving, and mood, the Chinese practitioner will attempt to devise a treatment plan that will help unblock your "stuck" qi, and bring your body back into balance.

Generally speaking, such a plan might include acupuncture (and possibly its related techniques of acupressure and massage) as well as herbal therapy, dietary advice, and qi-gong exercises. In general, the strategy for treating allergies in Chinese medicine involves cooling the inflammation, driving out the wind, drying up the dampness, and strengthening the underlying deficiencies. If your heart protector has been breached, the treatment will concentrate on strengthening what's known as the "circulation-sex" energy, using acupuncture needles with moxa.

As you can see, diagnosing your allergies and devising a healthy treatment plan for you according to Chinese traditions is a highly personal and complex process. Below are some general descriptions of treatment options, along with some basic prescriptions that may well apply to your particular condition.

ACUPUNCTURE, ACUPRESSURE, AND SHIATSU

There are over one thousand "acupoints" located throughout the body. The practitioner can stimulate these points with needles or with his hands to enhance the flow of qi through the body and thus restore health. Your doctor will show you, on a chart and on your body, exactly where along these channels your difficulty is located. The actual point of insertion or pressure depends on the site of your imbalance and the way in which your therapist wishes to influence qi.

Acupuncture needles are very long and very thin. Their insertion

ACUPUNCTURE AND CHINESE MEDICINE

should be nearly painless, although there is often a mild pinprick and tingling sensation as the energy pathways beneath the skin are breached. Often, moxibustion is used to warm and tone the body's qi before the needles are inserted. Moxa consists of special herbs derived from the mugwort plant and is gently heated either above or on a specific acupoint.

Acupuncture needles may be inserted to a depth of about one-fourth to two inches or more, depending on a variety of factors, including your size and the way that the practitioner wishes to influence the flow of qi. The practitioner always takes care to avoid blood vessels and major organs. The needles are left in place from a few seconds up to an hour; the average time is about 20 minutes. The type, extent, and location of your allergy symptoms, as well as the area of blocked qi, will determine how often and for how long you visit your acupuncturist. The average schedule is about once a week for several months, then once a month or so for maintenance.

For most cases of allergy, acupuncture would be both local (involving placing needles over the sinuses to open them up, for instance) and systemic (acupoints on what are known as the *tai yin* and *yang ming* meridians to clear up dampness and strengthen the lung, for instance, or on the lower *shao yang* gallbladder channel to eliminate wind).

Acupressure is different from acupuncture in that it uses finger pressure rather than needle insertion to stimulate acupoints. This method is especially helpful for those people who dislike or are afraid of needles, and it has the added comfort of physical, human touch. In addition, Chinese medical theory holds that a practitioner can transfer his or her own qi, or energy, to you through his or her hands, thus helping to heal you with touch. With a little training and guidance, you can learn to stimulate acupoints yourself and perform acupressure at home on your own.

One particular acupressure point known to help relieve allergies—even stop an attack before it begins—is the point in the center of the webbing of your hand, between your thumb and index finger. By gradually applying pressure to the point, angling the pressure toward the bone that connects with the index finger—then repeating the process on the other hand—you may find that you can arrest an allergy attack quickly.

A massage technique called shiatsu, developed in Japan, is another method of stimulating the flow of qi. The shiatsu therapist may use a combination of fingers, thumbs, elbows, knees, and feet to press acupoints, usually in a rhythmic pattern. He or she may also stroke your body as well as gently twist your spine and other joints to further relax you.

Acupuncture, acupressure, and shiatsu all have the same goal in mind: to ensure that the life-giving energy known as qi is moving unimpeded through your body. Qi-gong exercises, described a little later in this chapter, offer another way to stimulate qi and bring your body back into balance. In addition to these methods, Chinese medicine also uses herbs to nourish the body, mind, and spirit.

CHINESE HERBAL MEDICINE

The use of herbs is an essential part of traditional Chinese medicine. Herbs help to reorganize the body constituents (qi, blood, and body fluids) within the meridians and the internal organs, as well as help the body to cope with stress and other external forces. In general, Chinese herbal medicine involves using multiple herbs in combinations that have specific effects. Herbs are dispensed and can be used in many different forms, including pills, tinctures (alcohol-based solutions), or capsules. You might also use fresh herbs, either as teas or in food.

The practitioner of Chinese medicine that you visit will suggest certain herbs for you based on your particular problem and constitution. Although it would be counterproductive to attempt to prescribe herbs for you in this text, the following combinations are known to help relieve allergy symptoms. The practitioner will explain to you how much of these combinations to take, how to prepare them, and how often and when to use them.

For *allergic inflammation:* Xanthium, jade screen
For *stuffy noses and sinusitis: Pueraria* and magnolia
  combination

For asthma symptoms: minor blue dragon (which contains ephedra, known to dilate the bronchi)

For damp conditions: ginseng, cardamom, pinellia, and tangerine peel

For kidney deficient conditions: rehmannia, *Poria cocos*

For immune deficient conditions: astragalus, ganoderma mushroom

As is true for other aspects of allergy treatment within the Chinese medicine tradition, a practitioner will prescribe an herbal remedy for you only after carefully examining and evaluating your condition. Therefore, for you to attempt to self-medicate by purchasing and using these herbs on your own without guidance would be counterproductive.

QI-GONG EXERCISES

A third form of Chinese therapy is qi-gong, a literal translation of which is "energy exercises." Qi-gong builds qi and helps to move it freely around the body. The exercises work to cultivate inner strength, calm the mind, and help maintain the body's natural state of internal balance and harmony or, if upset, restore the balance.

There are several types of qi-gong. Some exercises are similar to calisthenics or isometric movements; others are like meditative stances, and still others involve the stimulation of acupressure points through massage. Breathing exercises attempt to bring the body into a state of relaxation and harmony. One such exercise involves the following steps:

1. While standing, breathe in through the nose, raising your arms above your head as you turn to your left side. At the same time, raise your right foot onto its toes.
2. Exhale through the nose and mouth, lowering your arms, and facing front.
3. Repeat the exercise, turning to the right side.
4. Perform the exercise six more more times to each side.
5. Perform the exercise seven times while facing front, raising your arms again above your head as you inhale. As you

exhale through your nose and mouth, lower your arms to
your sides.

6. Finally, stand with your arms at your sides, palms facing
   forward. Then inhale through your nose, moving your arms
   in a sideward arc until your palms meet over your head.
   Then exhale through the nose and mouth while lowering
   your arms to your sides. Repeat this phase six more times.

The basic qi-gong posture involves standing with the feet apart,
knees slightly bent, back straight, and the arms held in front of the
body. You are then to imagine that you are holding an imaginary "ball
of qi" in front of you. If this posture is maintained for a few minutes
to a half hour, you'll both improve your circulation and feel more
relaxed. Chinese medicine, with its emphasis on internal harmony and
self-care, is appealing to more and more Americans every day. Anxious to avoid the often painful, usually expensive, and almost always
futile mainstream treatments for arthritis, millions of men and women
find the ultimate goal of Chinese medicine—to bring internal harmony
and balance to the body and spirit—both immediately soothing and
ultimately motivating.

In Chapter 6, you'll learn about another system of medicine, one
developed in India, that also looks at health and healing from a holistic and natural perspective.

"With an eye made
quick by the power
of Harmony,
and the deep power
of joy, we see into
the life of things."

Wordsworth

Medicine from India

6

$\mathcal{A}$fter attending a lecture by an Ayurvedic practitioner and philosopher, Tony decided to visit an Ayurvedic doctor for treatment of allergies that had plagued him throughout most of his life. According to his mainstream doctor, who had performed skin testing, Tony was allergic to dust, pollen, trees, grasses, ragweed, and animal fur. Although tests had proved negative, Tony also believed he was allergic to wheat, corn, peanuts, and soy, and probably to other foods as well. In addition to standard hay fever symptoms (sneezing, stuffy nose, and coughing), his eyes burned, he experienced abdominal gas and bloating, and he was exceedingly restless.

Tony found a doctor trained in both Western and Ayurvedic medicine. On his first visit, the doctor took a standard medical history and performed a regular physical exam. During the exam, Tony was surprised that the doctor spent a great deal of time studying his tongue. She also took inordinate care in taking a series of pulses along his wrists. She asked if Tony had always been so slim (yes) and whether he tended to be sensitive to sounds, light, or even to emotional changes around him (also yes).

The doctor diagnosed Tony's allergic problems as a "primary vata disorder with a secondary pitta imbalance." She explained that within the Ayurvedic tradition there existed three biological humors, each present to a greater or lesser degree in every person and each with its own particular characteristics. The doctor explained that an imbalance of vata—the body type associated with the principle of air— made Tony's nervous and immune systems more sensitive, which led to allergies. His body reacted to foods that aggravated vata, like corn and soy. The pitta (fire) aspect of his disorder revealed itself in the inflammation of his eyes and sinuses.

The treatment began with a brief fast during which Tony drank a lemon tea made with honey. Although Tony had never been able to miss a meal without feeling weak, the fast actually seemed to help his symptoms. Then the doctor prescribed an "anti-vata" diet. The diet encouraged eating cooked rather than raw foods and eliminated most flour and yeast products, as well as other foods that expanded during cooking or preparation (since air made vata worse). The doctor told Tony to feel free to eat animal products, some whole cooked grains, nuts, and seeds, and certain cooked vegetables. Tony marveled at the detail in which the doctor and doctor's assistant went over his diet, as they even suggested he would do much better if he chose to eat with other people rather than by himself.

The next step in treatment involved performing a breathing exercise called lunar pranayama, in which Tony inhaled first through his left nostril (mentally saying the word "so"), then exhaled through his right nostril (saying "hum"). The doctor also showed him some simple yoga postures to practice, including the bow and the salute to the sun. To Tony, the strangest instruction of all involved a nasal and sinus cleansing ritual. Using a special container, called a netti pot, he first poured salted water into his sinuses, keeping his head back until the *sinuses became irrigated, then tilting his head forward to let them drain out. Though this procedure seemed odd at first, the doctor explained that Ayurveda considers the sinuses and colon "second skins" and therefore Tony should cleanse them just as he cleansed his skin.*

Finally, the doctor gave Tony herbs called Chyavan Prash and ashwaganda, as well as basil, gotu koa, calamus, and ginger. Tony also took a form of clarified butter called calamus ghee to rub around his nose, and an aromatic camphor-containing oil to dot around his forehead and temples each morning and evening. After faithfully following this program for a few months, Tony felt a great difference in the frequency and severity of his allergy attacks. Better still, he felt calmer than he had in years, his digestion was clearly better while he stayed on the diet, and he even felt more emotionally centered.

Like Tony, you may be searching for a new way to look at your body, your health, and your place in the universe and in nature. If you've been troubled by any allergy, you may want to explore Ayurveda, a tradition of health and healing that originated in ancient India.

In Sanskrit, the primary language of ancient India, Ayurveda means "knowledge of life." Indeed, far more than a compendium of medical treatments, Ayurveda represents a complete philosophy of life, living, and good health. Like its cousin traditional Chinese medicine, Ayurvedic medicine sees each individual person as an extension of the universe, and health as a state of balance within the body and between the body and the universe. In Ayurveda, as in most holistic forms of health and healing, there is no dividing line between body, mind, and spirit. Indeed, psychological and spiritual imbalances are just as apt to cause disease as physical imbalances. Your allergies, for instance, could stem from— or at least be exacerbated by—the fact that your life is too filled with stress or that you are unhappy in your relationships with others.

Treatment within the Ayurvedic tradition likewise attempts not to just relieve one or two symptoms in isolation, but instead works to bring the whole body back into balance. As Tony's case study shows, Ayurvedic medicine uses a combination of herbs, diet, cleansing rituals, and yoga.

The ABCs of Ayurvedic Philosophy

As you explore Ayurvedic principles in relation to your allergy problems, keep in mind that Ayurveda teaches that all of life—including disease and its symptoms—depends on and consists of learning and the development of self-knowledge. In this way, you might want to consider coming to terms with your allergies as an opportunity to reexamine your spiritual and physical state. By doing so, you would be working—spiritually and physically—to correct any internal imbalances and thus bring your body back into alignment with the energy of nature and the universe. Later in this chapter, we'll show you some of the ways Ayurvedic therapies may be used to treat allergies. In the meantime, here is a brief overview of Ayurvedic philosophy.

PRANA (THE LIFE FORCE) AND THE THREE DOSHAS

Known as "qi" in Chinese medicine, the life-providing energy in Ayurveda is called "prana." Prana is the animating power of life, providing vitality and endurance to each human being. Prana is also considered to be the power behind the healing process. Indeed, Ayurveda teaches that we each have a Divine Healer within us, nourished by prana, that if properly supported and directed can restore health and balance to the body.

Balance is a particularly important theme in Ayurvedic medicine, as it is in traditional Chinese medicine. In this Indian philosophy, balance and harmony are maintained by what is known as the *three doshas*, forces of energy that act upon body substances and organs. When the three doshas are balanced, the body functions harmoniously and in health. When they are out of balance, disease results.

The three doshas are called vata, pitta, and kapha. Vata represents movement and air; pitta, metabolism and heat; and kapha, structure. Within every cell of the body, these three operating principles must exist in proper balance for health to be maintained. Ayurveda teaches that a balance among the doshas will allow your physical, emotional, and intellectual qualities to function with vitality and energy.

According to Ayurvedic tenets, each individual has a specific body

type based on one of the three doshas. In essence, one of these qualities—movement, heat, or stability—predominates, helping to form
your unique personality and physiology. Your Ayurvedic body type
is like a blueprint outlining the innate tendencies built into your system. It helps to explain why you are able to consume lots of salt
without suffering any ill effects, while your sister's blood pressure
soars when she overloads on sodium. Or why eating certain foods
upsets your digestive system or causes you to break out in a rash, but
has no adverse consequences for your friend. Since a prime goal of
Ayurvedic medicine is to prevent disease from occurring in the first
place, understanding one's own dosha and practicing a lifestyle
designed to maintain dosha balance are essential. Furthermore, by
accurately identifying your body type, an Ayurvedic practitioner can
then diagnose and treat your condition more effectively.

Your body shape, your personality, and many other physical and
emotional attributes determine your dosha. Below are short descriptions of each type of dosha as it applies to body type:

Vata (pronounced "vah-tah") represents the force of movement
and air within your body. It activates the physical system and is
responsible for respiration and blood flow through the body. The seats
of vata—the places in the body from which it springs—are the large
intestine, pelvic cavity, skin, ears, and thighs. Organs associated with
vata include the brain (especially motor activity), the heart, and the
lungs. Vata is the dosha most associated with allergies, as well as with
arthritis and other musculoskeletal problems.

If you are predominately a vata body type, you tend to be rather
thin (like Tony), with prominent features and cool, dry skin. You tend
to speak rapidly and have an active, creative mind. You probably like
to keep irregular hours, and may be prone to feel anxious and worried. Vata's season is autumn—a dry, windy season during which vata
people often suffer from severe allergy flare-ups and other diseases of
the vata organs.

Pitta dosha governs the metabolic processes of cells. Organs associated with pitta include the blood, the brain (especially memory and
learning), hormones, liver, small intestine, and spleen. If you're a pitta

body type, you tend to have a medium build, thin hair, and warm, ruddy skin. Pittas are organized, work hard, and have very regular sleeping and eating patterns. Although generally warm and loving, a person with a predominately pitta dosha may also display quick bursts of temper. Pittas tend to suffer from acne, hemorrhoids, and ulcers, and may often feel warm and thirsty. The pitta season is summer, when the heat and bright light may aggravate pitta-related disorders, including allergy-related rashes, diarrhea, and inflammatory conditions.

Kapha is responsible for physical strength. Located in the chest, lungs, and spinal fluid, kapha holds together the structure of the body. Organs associated with kapha include the brain (information storage), joints, lymph, and stomach. If you have a predominately kapha body type, you tend to be heavyset, with cool, oily skin. Kaphas are often very relaxed and tolerant people, who are slow to anger and have a tendency to procrastinate. They sleep for long hours and may not eat for the physical reasons but rather for the emotional pleasure that food brings to them. Kapha types are especially prone to obesity as well as to illnesses of the kapha organs, such as allergies and sinus problems. The kapha season is winter, when the respiratory system is particularly susceptible to colds and congestion.

The Diagnostic Process

The Ayurvedic practitioner begins by asking you a series of questions about your personal life and habits as well as information about your allergy symptoms in particular. The practitioner will take note of not only *what* you say, but also the *way* you say it: the strength and sincerity (or lack thereof) in your voice may reflect your willingness to accept responsibility for your own health. The Ayurvedic practitioner will probably begin his physical examination of you by taking your pulse. In fact, he will listen to your pulse on 6 separate sites on the wrists—3 on the left and 3 on the right. Measuring the pulses informs the practitioner of the movement of energy—called prana—through the body, as well as the general health of each internal organ. Another important diagnostic tool used in Ayurvedic medicine, as well as in traditional Chinese medicine, is the examination of the tongue. Ayurvedic tradition divides the tongue into areas that reflect the different organs. The coating on the tongue indicates the amount and type of toxins in the organs. You may find it strange that he will want to smell and touch your skin during the exam; don't be alarmed, this is a perfectly natural part of the Ayurvedic diagnostic procedure.

Based on the results of these and other examination procedures, an Ayurvedic doctor will attempt to locate your physical and emotional strengths and weaknesses, as set forth by Ayurvedic tenets. We discuss some of those tenets in the section below.

The Ayurvedic Prescription

All treatment for allergies—indeed, for all illnesses and imbalances—involves the use of diet and nutrition, herbs, yoga exercises, meditation, massage, and breathing exercises. It is important to remember that Ayurvedic medicine does not treat any condition in isolation; and thus, the whole body must be brought into balance before a specific symptom, like itchy eyes, headaches, or congestion, can be alleviated.

Generally speaking, Ayurvedic medicine considers allergies to be an *ama* condition, one that involves the digestive system—even when food is not the direct trigger for an allergic response. According to this philosophy, a person with allergies is having trouble digesting certain foods, and this leads to a general breakdown of the entire body system and to allergic responses to otherwise benign substances.

PANCHAKARMA
The first step in your treatment may involve *panchakarma*, which is the process of detoxifying your body of impurities or toxins. Detoxification may consist of induced vomiting, enemas, blood cleansing (by bloodletting and using blood-thinning herbs)—even nasal douching

such as Tony performed—all under the strict and careful supervision of the Ayurvedic practitioner. Yoga, chanting, meditation, and lying in the sun for long periods make up another stage in the cleansing process.

A period of *tonification*, or enhancement, often follows. During tonification, you'll consume certain herbs and perform specific yoga and breathing exercises. At the same time, or perhaps as a next stage in the healing process, you'll spend a great deal of time meditating. Called *satvajaya*, the goal of this stage is to reduce your levels of psychological and emotional stress, as well as help you release negative emotions and ideas.

Once you've cleansed your body through this process, the practitioner is likely to devise a lifestyle plan to protect your body and keep it in balance. This plan involves eating the right foods and finding spiritual and physical energy through exercises known as yoga.

ALLERGY TIP

Many women are sensitive to the substances found in cosmetics. If you're one of them, try to use as few cosmetic products as possible. Avoid perfumes and scented products, instead opting for those labeled "unscented and hypoallergenic." Before using any new product, apply a small amount on the inside of your forearm and leave it on for 24 hours. If you experience any adverse reactions, don't use the product.

AN ALLERGY-FREE EATING PLAN

The Ayurvedic practitioner will devise an eating plan, based on your own specific needs and physiology. As you read in Tony's case history, such a diet is highly personal, and thus it would be impossible to guess what an Ayurvedic practitioner would find appropriate for your particular constitution and allergy problem.

Generally speaking, however, an antiallergy eating plan might include increasing foods that enhance the production of the immunoglobulin A (IgA). As you may remember from Chapter 2, this immunoglobulin resides primarily in the gastrointestinal tract and helps fight against harmful microbes that invade this part of the body. Herbs that help stimulate IgA production include ginger, garlic, onion, cayenne pepper, and black pepper. Any foods that use those herbs in their preparation might help to alleviate the underlying *ama* condition that may be causing your allergies. Furthermore, you might do well to try a rotation diet, such as that described in Chapter 4. In this way, you'll increase the variety of foods you eat while avoiding overwhelming your body with one substance. Again, however, a diet plan within this tradition is highly personal; if you are allergic to nightshade foods, for instance, eating lots of peppers would be quite counterproductive. You must work closely with your Ayurvedic practitioner to find an eating plan that is right for you.

YOGA: EXERCISE FOR THE BODY AND MIND

Yoga exercises help to stimulate and stretch your muscles and organs, as well as bring your mind and body into a deeper state of relaxation. There are dozens of yoga techniques and exercises and, in fact, several different schools of yoga, each one with a slightly different philosophy and emphasis. Indeed, the study of yoga in its fullest measure and many levels is a lifetime endeavor, one that, Ayurvedic tradition dictates, leads to true harmony and health.

Yoga poses, performed correctly and practiced regularly, will help you keep your body in balance and the muscles and tendons of your body supple and lithe. In his book *Perfect Health*, Deepak Chopra, M.D., describes a three-pronged yoga program that he prescribes to his patients. Called the "Three Dosha Exercises," it starts with an exercise called "The Sun Salutation," which is a complete Ayurvedic exercise that attempts to integrate your whole body, mind, and spirit. It also stretches and strengthens all of the major muscle groups and lubricates the joints while increasing blood flow throughout the body.

The Sun Salute consists of 12 postures that you should perform in a fluid sequence, one following directly after another. It is important that you keep breathing, deeply and regularly, throughout this exercise. Also keep in mind that the Sun Salutation, when performed correctly, is an invigorating exercise that takes energy and flexibility. Start slowly and don't strain your muscles trying to achieve positions your body isn't ready for.

The Sun Salutation (Surya Namaskar)

1. Stand up straight, feet together, with your fingers and palms together in front of your chest, your fingers pointing upward and your thumbs touching the chest. This is the traditional Indian gesture of respect or homage. If you like, think of the sun suffusing your body with energy.

2. As you inhale, raise your arms high and back, the palms facing forward. Let your head fall back, bending your spine gently backward from the waist.

3. As you exhale, bend forward from the waist and try to touch your hands to the floor beside your feet. Come as close as you can, but do not strain. Keep your knees slightly bent. Try to press your face to your thighs. If you can't quite reach the floor, bend your knees until you get your hands to the floor.

4. As you inhale and lift your head, stretch your right leg back and go down on your right knee. Your hands and left foot stay in position.

5. As you hold your breath, straighten your right leg and bring your left foot next to the right one. Your hands and toes are now supporting your body. From the back of your head to your heals should be a straight line. This is called the Wheelbarrow Pose.

6. As you exhale, bend your arms and lower your forehead, chest, and knees to the floor. Try to keep your pelvis and calves raised by pulling in your abdominal muscles and clenching your toes.

7. As you inhale, straighten your arms and raise your body up and back, keeping the pelvis and legs on the floor. Your back should form a gentle arc, with your chin pointing toward the ceiling.

8. As you exhale, bring your pelvis and hips up and bring your head between your hands. Your feet should stay flat on the floor, your palms should support your upper body, and your buttocks should form the highest point. Your body is now forming a triangle, with your hands and feet forming the base.

9. As you inhale, take a long step forward with your right foot, bringing it in line with your hands. At the same time, lower your left knee to the floor and bring your chest up and forward. (This is Position 4, only you're kneeling with your left knee instead of your right.)

10. As you exhale, assume Position 3 again by bringing your left foot forward beside your right foot, raising your hips, and straightening or nearly straightening your legs.

11. As you inhale, straighten up from the waist and swing your arms high and back, essentially repeating Position 2.

12. As you exhale, lower your arms to the side and stand up straight.

These 12 postures form the Sun Salutation. Once you've done it a few times, it should come naturally to you. Never bounce, strain, or rush during this exercise. Breathe deeply, feeling energy rush in every time you inhale and tension flee every time you exhale.

The Sun Salutation is just one of hundreds of yoga exercises. In *Natural Resources*, page 174, you'll find a list of books about yoga you might find of interest. In addition, you can look in your local phone book or ask at the YMCA for yoga classes being taught in your neighborhood.

Another common prescription for people interested in treating their bodies with Indian healing techniques is called balanced breathing or *pranayama*. This exercise involves learning to control and appreciate the act of taking oxygen in and releasing carbon dioxide and other toxins—including potential allergens like ragweed.

To perform a pranayama exercise that is particularly beneficial for those with allergies, gently close your right nostril with your thumb, then exhale and inhale once through your left nostril. Close your left nostril with the two middle fingers and exhale and inhale once with your right nostril. Continue alternating your breath between the two nostrils for five minutes. Remember to remain quiet, begin each breath on the *exhale* and finish on the *inhale*. Breathe naturally; do not feel the need to take deep breaths. You are simply learning to quiet your body and soul while bringing nourishment into your body.

As stated at the beginning of this chapter, Ayurvedic medicine is an ancient, complex, and multilayered system of health and healing. Its goal—to bring the body back into balance and harmony with nature and its natural state—is one that we should all strive to achieve. The closer you come to that ideal, the less likely you'll be to suffer from the effects of your allergies as often or as severely as you do today. If you are interested in pursuing Ayurvedic medicine in more depth, see *Natural Resources*, page 174. In the meantime, we now look to another way to treat allergies and other conditions, one that looks to the natural healing power of herbs.

"You don't fix people. What you're trying to do with human beings is to help them grow."

Lawrence LeShan

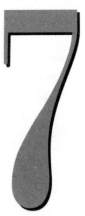

Herbal Medicine at Work

ℒoretta braced herself for another autumn during which her head would stay stuffy, her eyes would itch, her face would feel as if it were falling off, and her voice would sound like she spoke through pudding. For years, she'd taken allergy shots, which helped to alleviate some of her symptoms, but her doctor still kept her on daily antihistamines, decongestants, and eye drops. Tired of taking so many different medications, Loretta decided to seek the help of an herbalist, a woman with special skills and interests in aromatherapy.

The atmosphere in the aromatherapist's office was very relaxing and quieting. Loretta noticed a faint, very pleasant odor and found the lighting to be soft and comforting. The aromatherapist asked her to sit in a comfortable chair, which tilted back, and then asked her a series of questions about her allergic problems. In addition to

*recounting her symptoms, Loretta also admitted that she was under
extreme stress at work, and that her neck and shoulders felt chronically tight and sore.*

*The therapist then brought out several vials of scented oils and
placed them on the desk. She asked Loretta to smell two of them and
choose her favorite between them. Loretta chose an oil made of a mixture of lavender and eucalyptus. The therapist slowly rubbed a bit on
Loretta's temples, around her neck, into her jaw area, her temples, and
the back of her head. Then, using her thumbs, the therapist gently
massaged Loretta's cheekbones and across her sinuses. Loretta closed
her eyes and listened to soothing music in the background. Later
Loretta would tell a friend that it felt as if she had been transported to
the most relaxing place she could imagine.*

*Finally, the therapist massaged Loretta's neck and upper back,
explaining that the tight muscles in this area prevented proper lymph
drainage of the overworked sinuses. She finished by having Loretta
inhale a different essential oil, one containing essences of lemon and
thyme. She sent Loretta home with a tincture and instructed her to place
some in hot water and inhale it several times per day, massaging her
sinuses as she did so. Loretta left the office feeling healthier and more
balanced than she had in many years, and her nose and eyes felt clear.*

*Loretta administered her treatments at home as directed and paid
regular visits to the aromatherapist during allergy season. Although
she still used some medications occasionally, she experienced the easiest, healthiest allergy season she could remember.*

The Healing Power of Herbs

As foreign as it may seem to those of us accustomed to modern
pharmaceuticals, herbal medicine has formed an integral part of
every culture in history. Even modern mainstream medicine is inti-
mately linked to herbal traditions: trees, shrubs, or other plants and

natural materials form the basis of approximately 25 percent of all prescription drugs in the United States today. The rest of the world uses herbal medicine even more often. Europeans, for example, spend more than $6 billion per year on herbal medications. In addition man-made versions of natural plants and organic compounds comprise another huge segment of the pharmaceutical market. Today, however, more and more people are looking to traditional herbal medicine and its cousin aromatherapy as they search for more healthful, natural ways of healing.

Like other forms of alternative therapy, herbal medicine and aromatherapy attempt not to cure disease per se, but rather to help the body remain in, or return to, the state of balance we know of as health. In attempting to make this happen, herbalists tend to explore lifestyle and dietary habits with their patients in order to develop a treatment plan far more individualized and personal than most mainstream physicians care to do.

Although each person who visits an herbalist or aromatherapist will likely emerge with a different prescription (even for the very same complaint), there are some generalities that can be made about possible remedies for allergies: an herbalist might recommend herbs to help eliminate toxins and allergens, others to bolster the immune system, still others that work to treat specific symptoms like congestion, upset stomach, or itchy skin. As for an aromatherapist, she might recommend a variety of essential oils for generally the same purposes: to ease respiratory or gastrointestinal distress while strengthening the body as a whole.

At a first appointment with an herbalist, you should expect the practitioner to take a complete medical history. Among the most important topics discussed will be the exact nature of your symptoms and triggers, and any past medical treatment you've had for your allergies. Based on what the herbalist discovers during the exam, she would then prescribe one or more natural medications aimed at strengthening your underlying constitution while alleviating your symptoms.

Herbal Medicine: Nature's Pharmacy

In general, herbal medicines work in much the same way as conventional pharmaceutical drugs. Herbs contain a large number of naturally occurring substances that work to alter the body's chemistry in order to return it to its natural state of health. Unlike purified drugs, however, plants and other organic material contain a wide variety of substances and, hence, less of any one particular active component. This attribute makes herbs far less potentially toxic to the body than most pharmaceutical products. Another benefit of natural herbs is that they tend to contain combinations of substances that work together to restore balance to the body with a minimum of side effects. The plant meadowsweet is a good example: it contains compounds similar to the ones used in aspirin that act as antiinflammatories. These compounds, called salicylates, often irritate the stomach lining. Unlike commercially prepared aspirin, however, meadowsweet also contains substances that soothe the gastric lining and reduce stomach acidity, thus providing relief from pain while protecting the stomach from irritation.

Herbs of all types are available in many forms including:

Whole herbs: Plants or plant parts are dried and either cut or powdered to be used as teas or as cooking herbs.

Capsules and tablets: Increasingly popular with consumers, capsules and tablets allow people to consume herbs quickly and without tasting them.

Extracts and tinctures: Extracts and tinctures are made by grinding the roots, leaves, and flowers of an herb and immersing them in a solution of alcohol and water for a period of time. The alcohol works to extract the maximum amount of active ingredients from the herb and acts as a preservative.

Poultices and ointments: Ground herbs form the base of external applications to be placed directly on your skin. Poultices are hot packs applied to the skin, made by mixing ground herbs with hot water, placing them in a muslin bag, then applying them to the sore joint or muscle. An ointment is a cream or salve with an herbal base that you can buy in health food stores or through your herbalist.

Herbs Used to Treat Allergies

A prescription for an herbal remedy is apt to be quite personal and individual, based on your particular symptoms, habits, and needs. Listed below are some of the herbs prescribed most often for men and women with allergies.

TO REDUCE MUCUS ACCUMULATION

Goldenseal *(Hydrastis canadensis)*. Also known as yellow root, goldenseal dries up and soothes the mucous membranes throughout the body. This quality makes it useful in alleviating congestion and excess mucus, both in the respiratory system and in the digestive tract.

Prescription and preparation: Goldenseal is usually sold as capsules (taken 2 to 5 times a day) and as a tincture (½ to 1 teaspoon a day). You also can buy it in powdered form, from which you can make a tea by pouring a cup of boiling water over about ½ to 1 teaspoon of the powder (taken twice a day).

Red Sage *(Salvia officinalis)*. Red sage is a classic remedy for inflamed and congested mucous membranes. It may be used internally and as a mouthwash (if your throat and mouth are also sore).

Prescription and preparation: You can use about 1 teaspoon of dried red sage leaves to make a tea to drink up to 3 times a day. Red sage tincture is also available. You can take about 2 to 4 milliliters 3 times per day.

TO REDUCE INFLAMMATION

Cayenne *(Capsicum minimum)*. Cayenne, which we as Americans know as hot red pepper, is one of the most useful herbal remedies available. Its active ingredient, capsaicin, is a strong antiinflammatory and thus helps to soothe burning nasal passages, bronchial tubes, and lungs. Cayenne is also a good digestive tonic and benefits the heart and circulation. It is rich in vitamin C and other powerful antioxidants.

Prescription and preparation: Cayenne is readily available in powdered form and can be used in food, drunk as a tea (a cup of boiling water over ½ to 1 teaspoon of cayenne), and taken as a tincture (0.25 to 1 milliliter 3 times a day).

Yarrow (*Achillea millefolium*). A powerful antiinflammatory, yarrow is useful in treating fevers. It also reduces blood pressure, stimulates digestion, and reduces swelling of bronchial tissue.

Prescription and preparation: You can use dried yarrow leaves to make a tea, or you can consume it in tincture form (about 2 to 4 milliliters 3 times a day).

TO STRENGTHEN THE IMMUNE SYSTEM

Astragalus (*Astragalus membranaceus*). This ancient Chinese herb, is still used to increase resistance to disease. It has a warming effect on the body and soothes the digestive tract and other organs.

Prescription and preparation: Astragalus is most commonly available in commercial form as capsules (1 400-milligram capsule up to 3 times daily) and tinctures (1 teaspoon 3 times daily).

Echinacea (*Echinacea angustifolia*). Also known as purple coneflower, this plant is a traditional Native American remedy known to have extraordinary immune-boosting qualities. Many clinical and laboratory studies document the ability of echinacea to strengthen the body's tissues and protects you from invasive germs and allergens.

Prescription and preparation: You can buy echinacea in any number of different forms: capsules (1 capsule up to 3 times a day), tinctures (1 teaspoon up to 3 times a day), and extracts (mix 15 to 30 drops in water or juice and take up to 4 times a day).

Remember, herbs *are* drugs and may have serious side effects if not taken properly. It is best to devise an herbal prescription plan with a trained professional. That said, let's take a look at a related system of natural medicine that also uses plants to heal: aromatherapy.

The Healing Power of Scent

On your way to work one morning, you catch a whiff of lavender perfume wafting from the open windows of a neighborhood pharmacy. Almost immediately, you are awash in pleasant memories of your childhood: transported back in time and space to your grandmother's home, where lavender sachets lined linen drawers and scented sheets covered the guest bed, you feel as warm and secure as you did when you were 9 years old. By the time you arrive at your office, you feel more calm and relaxed than you have in weeks. If a doctor were to take your blood pressure, he might even find it lower than usual.

Although this example may not apply directly to you, no doubt you've experienced something similar. Perhaps the odor of a particular food evokes a feeling of comfort or the scent of certain flowers gives you energy. This strong connection between scent, emotion, and memory has led to a revival of an ancient form of medical intervention known as aromatherapy.

A French chemist named René-Maurice Gattefossé coined the term "aromatherapy" in 1937 after badly burning his hand during a laboratory experiment in his family's perfume factory. Knowing that lavender was used in medicine for burns, he plunged his hand into a vat of pure lavender oil used to make perfume. After noticing that his hand healed very quickly, Gattefossé began to explore the healing powers of other essential oils.

Essential oils, composed of the plant's most volatile constituents, are extracted from plants through a process of steam distillation or cold pressing. To derive pure essential oils, no other chemicals or substances should be used during the extraction process, since they would disrupt the natural organic composition of plant material. Indeed, each essential oil is made up of several different organic molecules that, working together, give the oil its unique perfume as well as its particular therapeutic qualities.

Like the plants and herbs from which they are extracted, some essential oils are known to have antiviral and antibacterial properties and thus can be used to treat infections such as herpes simplex, skin and bowel infections, and the flu. Perhaps the most common aromatherapy uses oil derived from the eucalyptus plant. When inhaled, eucalyptus works to restore health to the respiratory system by acting as an antibacteria and antiviral agent as well as an expectorant—a special boon to people with allergies who have respiratory symptoms.

Other therapeutic oils ease the antiinflammatory response in the body while boosting the immune system, making these oils especially useful in treating allergies. In addition, there are a number of oils that have profound effects on the central nervous system. Stress overstimulates the sympathetic nervous system and forces the muscles to tense up and, eventually, to shorten. Certain essential oils, when inhaled, can help to bring your nervous system into balance and thus reduce the negative effects stress may have on the body.

USING AROMATHERAPY

Essential oils are delicate, highly concentrated essences of plants. The quantity of plant material needed to make even a small amount of essential oil is enormous: to make an ounce of lavender oil, for instance, requires about 12 pounds of fresh lavender flowers. Fortunately, only a very small amount of oil is needed to have therapeutic effects.

You can buy essential oils in their pure form or already diluted with another base oil, usually made from olives, soy, or almonds. In addition, herbs that "fix" the scents are added, so that the potency of the mixture is maintained over time. Combining essences with base oils does not change their chemical composition, but will help to reduce their potential toxicity to the skin or internal tissue.

Although it is possible to make your own essential oils with a homemade still, most people choose to purchase prepared oils from health food stores or mail order companies. However, it is important that you make sure that the essential oils you use are just that: essential, meaning that their original chemical compositions were not altered in any way during the extraction process. Make sure that when you buy oils the word "essential" is used on the label and that you buy your oils from a reputable dealer. For more information, see *Natural Resources*, page 174.

In general, there are two main ways to use essential oils:

As Inhalants. Simply breathing in the odors and minute particles of plant material will help bring your body back into balance.

There are several equally effective methods of inhaling essential oils:

Aroma lamps: Putting a few drops of oil on a light bulb or burning a candle under a cup that has drops of oil in it will volatize the oil into the atmosphere, making your whole environment rich with soothing aroma.

Diffusers: Mechanical devices disperse essential oils into the air.

Facial saunas: Pour boiling water into a bowl, then add a few drops of essential oil. Drape a towel over your head and lean over the bowl so that the towel encloses both head and bowl. The essences are thus absorbed both through the skin and through the membranes of the nasal passages.

As Topical Applications. When prepared properly with base oils (a process completed before you purchase them), essential oils may be safely and effectively applied directly to the skin.

Bath oils: Adding a few drops of an essential oil to bathwater both adds to the relaxing atmosphere and allows the oils to seep into the skin. Warm baths are also helpful in easing sore, stiff joints.

Massage oils: Oils can be massaged into the face, back, chest, or any part of the body. Loretta, the allergy sufferer you met at the beginning of the chapter, derived a great deal of benefit from essential oil massage, both in the therapist's office and at home.

Poultice: An age-old way of relieving congestive inflammation, such as that which may develop with chronic pain and stiffness, poultices are made by moistening raw herbs and applying them directly to the affected areas.

Most people can use aromatherapy oils safely. In order to ensure that you do not suffer an adverse reaction, follow these simple tips:

Perform a patch test. Before you use any essential oil on your skin, whether in the bath, as a liniment, or as a massage oil, make sure you first perform a patch test. To do so, wash about a two-inch-square area on your forearm and dry it carefully. Apply a tiny drop of the essential oil, diluting it with an equal part of a bland oil, like olive oil. Then place a piece of gauze over the area and wait 24 hours. If no irritation occurs, feel free to use the oil in the future. If you develop a rash or are otherwise made uncomfortable, look for an alternate oil for your symptoms. A patch test is especially important if you have allergies or if your skin is particularly sensitive.

Check with your doctor. If you are pregnant, check with both your obstetrician and your alternative practitioner before using any essential oils. Do not take essential oils internally unless you first discuss the matter thoroughly with your practitioner. Some oils are highly toxic if swallowed.

Watch out for your eyes. Keep essential oils out of eyes.

Protect essential oils. Store essential oils in dark glass or metal bottles and protect them from light and heat.

Aromatherapy and Allergies

The following is a list of essential oils that may help to ease the symptoms of your allergies, by reducing the irritating process of inflammation, by boosting the immune system, or by relieving the stress and tension that trigger and aggravate your allergic reaction.

Please note that this is a highly subjective list and that many other oils may work just as well, if not better, depending on your own individual constitution and needs. That's why it is important that you visit an herbalist trained in aromatherapy to learn more about how to apply this ancient art to your particular health problem.

Chamomile. The leaves, flowers, and even roots of this yellow daisylike flower are used in a variety of different ways to treat several kinds of diseases and conditions. Aromatherapists use chamomile oil for its ability to soothe an aggravated nervous system. You can dab a drop or two of chamomile oil on your temples, make a hot compress with chamomile oil and hot water on a terrycloth washcloth and place against an aching joint, or you can sprinkle oil in a diffuser and inhale it all day long.

Lavender (*Lavandula officinalis*). Probably best known as a perfume, this herb has many valuable medicinal qualities as well. Gently rubbing lavender oils on your temples when you are under particular stress or when you're experiencing an allergy flare-up will certainly give you a lift.

Eucalyptus Oil (*Eucalyptus* spp.). One of the best remedies for congestion of the lungs and nasal passages, eucalyptus oil is especially soothing when mixed with rosemary oil.

Rosemary Oil (*Rosmarinus officinalis*). Rosemary oil, distilled from the tops, leaves, and smaller twigs of the rosemary plant, may be used as a massage oil when added to an olive or vegetable oil, and/or mixed with eucalyptus oil. It may also be inhaled by any of the methods mentioned above (diffuser, aroma lamp, facial sauna). According to herbal tradition, inhaling rosemary oil helps to increase sensitivity to situations, develop a better memory, and strengthen the power of the pineal gland—the gland that secretes melatonin, one of the body's most powerful natural sleep-aids.

Again, although these remedies are generally considered quite safe, it is important that you seek the advice of an herbalist or other health practitioner experienced in the use of herbs for medicinal purposes. Herbs are indeed drugs, and they have the power to cause unwanted effects and side effects if taken carelessly. That said, anyone suffering from a long-term, chronic illness like allergies is likely to find the use of herbs a welcome substitute or addition to other remedies to relieve pain and stress.

In the next chapter, we introduce another alternative approach to treating allergies, one that concentrates on the proper alignment of your spine and musculoskeletal system as the key to good health.

"They knew that

the body could

not be cured

without the mind."

Socrates

(about the Thracians)

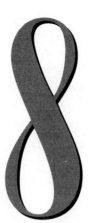

Spinal and Cranial Manipulation: Chiropractic and Osteopathy

James experienced sinus headaches several times a day, and they were actively interfering with his ability to work. As a salesman, he had to be "on" all the time, but his throbbing headache made it difficult for him to convince anyone of anything. When he took medication, it dulled his headache but also dulled his thinking. In desperation, he asked friends for advice. Someone referred him to an osteopath who practiced a technique known as cranial osteopathy.

James had heard of a massage practitioner who used something called craniosacral therapy, *which worked to help the movement of fluid in the brain and spinal column. The osteopath explained that the two techniques were similar, but that only physicians (usually osteopaths) practiced cranial osteopathy. The doctor explained that mainstream physicians thought that the bones of the head were immobile, but that osteopaths believe that the skull bones actually have some range of movement between them. A trained osteopath could feel the movement as a pulsing when he placed his or her hands upon the skull during an examination. When something like a sinus inflammation from allergies occurred, with pressure from sinusitis, it affected the rhythmic movement of these bones, and prevented the inflammation from healing well.*

The doctor had James lie down, and then he placed his hands on James's head. For a long time, James felt like nothing was happening, but soon began to feel very relaxed and noticed that his nose was clear for the first time in days. The doctor gave James instructions to stay away from dairy foods and suggested he come again for a series of six manipulation sessions. During the next week, James felt that there was a release of some of the chronic pressure in his sinuses. By the sixth session, James was a believer. His headaches, while still present, were not as bothersome, and he was able to get through a sales conference in top form.

Making Adjustments

It may seem strange to you to see a chapter about spinal and cranial manipulation in a book about allergies. After all, you've probably heard about chiropractic and osteopathy only in connection with back pain or other musculoskeletal problems, not with conditions involving other systems of the body. In this chapter, we'll show you that the theory behind spinal manipulation encompasses far more than the bones of the spine and skull and the muscles attached to them.

Spinal manipulation therapy is just what it sounds like: treatment of medical disorders that involves readjusting the vertebrae of the spine and, in some practices, the suture spaces of the skull. The spinal column is made up of 33 bones, called vertebrae, that surround the spinal cord, which is a sheaf of nerve tissue reaching from the base of the brain to the upper part of the lower back. Between adjoining vertebrae are pairs of spinal nerves that extend to every part of the body. Should the vertebrae become misaligned—through trauma, stress, or a chemical imbalance—pressure is placed on the nerves in the affected area. Should that area be involved with the kidney area of the body, for instance, the adrenal glands may not receive the nourishment and nerve impulses they need to produce enough adrenaline, thereby worsening the allergic response.

Two alternative schools of medicine, chiropractic and osteopathy, consider the spine and the nervous system that springs from it to be the center of all health in the body. Today, more than 94 percent of all manipulative care is delivered by chiropractors, 4 percent by osteopaths, and the remaining 2 percent by general practitioners and orthopedic surgeons. Let's take them one at a time.

Chiropractic Technique

Chiropractic is a word derived from the Greek *cheir*, meaning "hand," and *praktikis*, meaning "practical." Although spinal adjustment has been practiced by nearly every culture in history, a self-educated healer named Daniel David Palmer developed the modern school of chiropractic in 1895. Palmer's first patient was a janitor who had been deaf for almost 20 years. By bringing the man's spine back into alignment through massage and pressure, Palmer restored his hearing. Palmer believed that the janitor had lost his hearing because an injury had damaged his spine, preventing the central nervous system from delivering messages to and from the brain and ear. Palmer also believed that the body has an innate ability to heal itself, an ability controlled by the central nervous system. If the spine becomes misaligned, then, the body can no longer restore balance on its own to any part of the body.

Chiropractic therapy centers on restoring proper balance and structure to the spinal column and joints and, by doing so, restoring proper working order to the nervous system that radiates from the spinal cord to the organs and tissues of the body. When the vertebrae are properly aligned and the spine remains flexible, nerve impulses from the brain can travel freely along the spinal cord and to the all the organs and tissues of the body.

By keeping the spine in alignment through regular visits to the chiropractor, so the theory holds, you will allow all the systems of your body to work in harmony. Should you have an allergic reaction occur, you'll be less likely to suffer a severe attack if nerve impulses and the physiological responses they engender flow unimpeded. Furthermore, by keeping the nervous system in good working order, you'll be allowing your body to function well as a whole, and thus be able to heal itself of most ailments. According to theory, then, chiropractic should be seen as both treatment for disease and a method of preventing disease.

CHIROPRACTIC DIAGNOSIS AND TREATMENT

Your evaluation with a chiropractor begins the minute you walk through the office door. The chiropractor will pay just as much careful attention to the way you walk, stand, and sit as he will to any x-ray or other diagnostic test. After watching the way you move, the chiropractor will ask you questions about your symptoms and past medical history. (In fact, because a chiropractor is not a medical doctor, it is extremely important that you rule out any medical problems that could be causing your allergies before you visit a chiropractor.) He will ask about your allergy symptoms and what tends to bring them on. You both will spend a great deal of time assessing your work environment, relationships, exercise habits, and diet to see how each might contribute to your problem.

Following this discussion, the chiropractor will administer an orthopedic exam, during which special attention is paid to the range of movement of your spine and limbs. He'll probably ask you to bend forward, backward, and sideways, and to rotate your spine. Then he'll perform a neurological examination, including reflex testing, to assess nerve function. The chiropractor may feel the spine and various other joints with his or her hands (palpation) to further assess mobility and alignment. Under certain circumstances, you may require x-rays so that the chiropractor can confirm a diagnosis.

Once your chiropractor decides where your particular misalignment—or *subluxation,* as disturbances in the spine are called in chiropractic—occurs, the chiropractic adjustment begins. Depending on what kind of subluxation the chiropractor finds in your spine, he may choose to perform an *active* manipulation, in which you'll stretch your body in a certain way yourself, or a *passive* manipulation, in which the chiropractor assists your movement, helping to stretch the spine past its range of passive movement using his hands. Another process, known as the *high-velocity thrust,* involves the chiropractor placing his hands on a particular vertebral area and then thrusting forward with a certain amount of force and speed.

One of the most common chiropractic manipulations used to alleviate allergies involves a manipulation of the cervical vertebrae, the vertebrae located in the upper part of your back and neck. By manipulating these bones and the nerves encased within them, the chiropractor attempts to provide energy to the sympathetic nervous system while helping to clear the sinuses and nasal passages.

Your particular needs and physical constitution form the basis upon which the chiropractor determines the type of adjustment and the technique used. Do not be alarmed if your body makes some cracking or hissing noises during treatment: these are signs that the bones are moving and gases within the joints are being released. Although chiropractic should never be painful, you may feel a certain pressure and achiness during and for a few days following your first few treatments.

Appointments usually last from 30 to 60 minutes. Most chiropractors will suggest one or two visits a week for a couple of weeks, then one every three weeks for maintenance. Generally speaking, the more entrenched and long-standing your allergic problem is, the longer it will take to resolve it. On the other hand, if chiropractic is going to work for you, you should see a substantial improvement in symptoms in about a month to six weeks.

FINDING A QUALIFIED CHIROPRACTOR

Chiropractic now ranks as the second-largest primary health care field in the world, with more than 18 million Americans visiting a chiropractor every year, a great majority of them seeking relief from stubborn, chronic back pain. There are more than 50,000 chiropractors practicing in the United States today.

Although not medical doctors, chiropractors are among the more highly trained alternative caregivers, requiring at least six years of undergraduate and postgraduate training at colleges accredited by an agency officially recognized by the United States Department of Education. Chiropractors become licensed in all 50 states after passing rigorous state-controlled examinations.

To find a qualified chiropractor, your first step might be to ask your own family doctor. In recent years, chiropractors have been able to form a cordial working relationship with much of the mainstream medical community. Also, feel free to ask your friends and acquaintances for referrals—word of mouth is one of the best ways to find a qualified and caring health professional—or check with the American Chiropractic Association or the International Chiropractors Association.

ALLERGY TIP

Purchase an electronic air cleaner if inhalants cause you allergy problems. These cleaners come with a charged filter that attracts molds, house dust, and pollen from the air. The best models use high-efficiency particulate air (HEPA) filters. Some air cleaners fit on forced-air heating systems; some are room-sized stand-alone units.

Osteopathy

Although this branch of Western medicine remains new to many Americans, osteopathy was founded by a traditional American physician, Andrew Taylor Still, more than 120 years ago. Dr. Still modeled his philosophy of medicine on the theories postulated by the Greek father of medicine, Hippocrates. Hippocrates believed that the body could cure itself and that a doctor should be trained to study aspects of health, rather than symptoms of illness, in order to understand and treat disease.

In addition, Dr. Still postulated that the body can function properly only if blood and nerve impulses are allowed to flow throughout the body unimpeded. If your spine or another joint comes out of alignment and blocks blood and nerve flow, disease and pain may result. And because the musculoskeletal system is the body's largest energy user, tension or restriction in this system can deplete the rest of the body of its energy and thus result in illness.

Cranial osteopathy is a specific branch of osteopathy that concentrates on the movement of cerebrospinal fluid within and surrounding the craniosacral system—that is, the system composed of the head, the spine, and the tailbone and including the brain, the spinal cord, and the cerebrospinal fluid that bathes the brain and spinal cord. If the flow of cerebrospinal fluid becomes disrupted for any reason, disease may result. According to cranial osteopathic theory, there is a rhythmic motion in the craniosacral system created by the movement of the tiny sutures of the skull. The goal of the cranial osteopath is to remove any stress and pressure from between the cranial bones, thus allowing the cerebrospinal fluid to flow more freely to all parts of the body.

Of all the medical specialties, osteopathy is considered to be the most holistic, tending as it does to treat the whole person rather than one set of symptoms or health concerns. Osteopathic treatment centers on restoring balance and order to the musculoskeletal system— and thus to your whole body—through spinal manipulation. Attention is also paid to diet, exercise, and other habits that may be affecting your health.

YOUR OSTEOPATHIC EXAM AND TREATMENT

Unlike chiropractors, osteopaths are licensed medical doctors who receive extra training in spinal manipulation and the musculoskeletal system in general. Osteopaths are able to perform extensive diagnostic tests, prescribe drugs, and perform surgery. Although most osteopaths are general practitioners, some may have chosen training in a main-stream specialty, such as gynecology, pediatrics, or surgery.

Your first appointment with an osteopath should be quite similar to one with a mainstream physician, with a few notable exceptions. First, she will most likely spend a great deal of time discussing your general health, your medical history, your symptoms, and your personal habits. Second, she will pay special attention to the way you sit, stand, and walk, and may ask you to perform special exercises to see how your body moves. Asymmetry, a condition in which one side of your body is being held off-center and thus placing stress on part of the body, is one condition osteopaths attempt to identify. Osteopaths also look for any abnormal increase or decrease to the normal curve of the spine.

Third, the osteopath will probably spend far more time touching your body, particularly your spine and lower back, than a mainstream physician might. She will feel for temperature and texture changes of the skin, areas of muscular tension, tenderness or swelling, and nerve reflexes. Once the osteopath locates the source of your problem, she will help you work out a treatment plan. In most cases of allergies, this will involve the following:

Medication or Surgery. Because osteopathy blends conventional with alternative approaches, osteopaths may be more likely than other holistic practitioners to recommend mainstream medical solutions. On the other hand, they are more apt to suggest trying alternative approaches at their disposal before attempting more radical solutions.

Manipulation. Like chiropractors, osteopaths use their hands—and sometimes gentle currents of electricity or ultrasound technology—to release tension from muscles and restore proper alignment to the spine and other joints. Cranial manipulation, such as that practiced on James at the beginning of this chapter, involves very gentle manipulation of the skull.

Relaxation Techniques. By prescribing specially designed meditation and visualization exercises, such as those described in Chapter 10, osteopaths help you to maintain your body's structural integrity by preventing stress and tension from disrupting your immune system.

Breathing Exercises. Deep breathing exercises are meant to help bring life-enhancing oxygen and other nutrients to all the tissues of the body.

Posture Correction. Borrowing from a variety of bodywork techniques, including some of those described in Chapter 12, osteopaths attempt to correct postural imbalances that may be exacerbating your allergies or that have occurred when your body tenses up during an allergy attack. By teaching you how to use your body in a more efficient and less stressful way, osteopaths hope to help you reduce stress and tension.

Nutritional Guidance. Because osteopathy is essentially a holistic approach to health and healing, your osteopath will assess the state of your diet, help determine if a food allergy is involved, and then help you to develop an eating and nutritional plan that will keep you healthy and fit.

FINDING A QUALIFIED OSTEOPATH

Today, more than 35,000 osteopaths practice in the United States. The training they receive in the 15 osteopathic medical colleges blends conventional medical and surgical techniques with osteopathic manipulative techniques. Medical doctors (M.D.'s) who are also osteopaths carry the title Doctor of Osteopathy or D.O. and are listed in the telephone book under Physicians and Surgeons. You may also seek information about locating an osteopath through the American Academy of Osteopathy or the American Osteopathic Association.

Both chiropractic and osteopathy are largely based on Western medical traditions. In the next chapter, we explore an approach to health and healing known as homeopathy, one that embraces some concepts and techniques that may be unfamiliar to you.

"You may honestly feel grateful that homeopathy survived the attempts of the allopathists to destroy it."

Mark Twain

9

Homeopathy and Allergies

$\mathcal{D}$erived from the Greek word *homoios* (meaning "similar") and *pathos* (meaning "suffering), homeopathy is a holistic form of medicine, one that views the individual as a totality of interdependent parts, with no separation between the mental and physical realms. Since Dr. Samuel Hahnemann, a German physician, developed homeopathy in the 1800s, this discipline has offered a striking alternative to Western medical techniques and theories, especially for those people who suffer from a chronic condition like allergy.

Until recently, homeopathy has remained a relatively obscure branch of alternative medicine, at least in the United States. Today, however, more and more Americans are flocking to the increasing numbers of homeopaths practicing in cities and towns across the country—including in an increasing number of health maintenance organizations (HMOs). Homeopathic remedies now earn more than $165 million a year in sales, mostly from health food stores and neighborhood pharmacies.

Perhaps most important, a number of homeopaths have published studies in mainstream medical journals that point to the effectiveness of this still controversial treatment option. A 1994 study published in the British journal *The Lancet,* for instance, is of special interest to people with allergies: it found that a homeopathic remedy called arsenicum album (described later in this chapter) brought relief to 28 men and women allergic to dust mites.

The Homeopathic Philosophy

Samuel Hahnemann was a deeply spiritual man who believed that a physician's primary role should be as a catalyst, that true healing could not take place by simply administering drugs that would, in essence, override the body's natural processes. Homeopaths still espouse that point of view. In the case of allergies, for instance, homeopaths interpret the symptom of a runny nose as a positive and necessary flow of waste products from the body in order to dispel offending substances. Orthodox medicine, on the other hand, views the same symptom as inherently negative, requiring suppression. Unfortunately, by suppressing the symptom by taking antihistamines, an individual ends up retaining substantial amounts of the very substances that trigger the runny nose in the first place.

Dr. Hahnemann also believed that we each contain within us a "vital force," a life power animating and ruling the body, keeping it in balance and health. Disease occurs when a disturbance of this vital force takes place. Homeopathy considers symptoms of disease to be the external evidence of the vital force's internal attempts to bring the body back to a state of balance—the runny nose, for instance, ridding the body of irritating, disruptive allergens.

To a homeopath, a "disease" consists of the symptoms produced by the body in its own efforts to heal itself. And to encourage that healing process, homeopaths administer tiny doses of substances that will trigger the body to produce those very symptoms. This principle is known as Hahnemann's *Law of Similars,* or "like cures like." By making symptoms worse, a remedy strengthens the body's own power to heal itself. In fact, homeopathic theory holds that any therapy that attempts to suppress the free flow of symptoms—such as the use of antihistamines, decongestants, or other drugs—will actually prolong the underlying disturbance, since it prevents the body from being able to heal itself.

Another theory of homeopathic medicine is known as the *Law of Infinitesimals.* First developed by Dr. Hahnemann in order to reduce the side effects of often potentially toxic chemicals, this theory states that the smaller the dose of medicine, the greater its potency and its effect on the body's vital force. Homeopathic remedies are extracts derived by soaking plant, animal, mineral, or other biological material in alcohol or water to form what is known as the "mother tincture." This tincture is again diluted with alcohol in ratios of 1 part tincture to 10 or 100 parts of alcohol, shaken vigorously, then diluted again.

This process of shaking and diluting, repeated several times, is known as "succussion." Many researchers believe that through succussion the vital energy of a substance is transferred to the tincture. Therefore, the more times the solution is passed through succussion, the more potent the remedy, although there appears to be no trace of the original herb or mineral left. Finally, the resulting solution is added to tablets, usually made of sugar (sucrose and lactose). Homeopathic remedies are dispensed in either drop or pill form.

Obtaining a Homeopathic Prescription

Homeopaths write prescriptions only after carefully evaluating an individual's particular set of symptoms as well as her physical and emotional makeup. Indeed, a session with a homeopath may be a unique experience for those of us accustomed to Western medicine's approach to diagnosis and treatment. A homeopath will spend much more time talking to you about your symptoms and lifestyle factors, and look more carefully at your demeanor, personality, and coloring, than would a mainstream physician.

In fact, the way that diseases or conditions like allergies are treated by a homeopath depends entirely on your particular pattern of symptoms. And because homeopaths consider mental and emotional disturbances to be more serious and telling than physical symptoms, a homeopath will spend a great deal of time talking to you about your moods, the level of stress in your life, and any emotional or psychological upsets you've experienced recently or in the past. Interestingly enough, the symptoms that first bring you to the homeopath (called *common symptoms* in homeopathy) are rarely the most important symptoms when it comes to selecting a remedy. Instead, homeopaths give *general symptoms,* which include your state of mind and mood, more weight in determining a treatment. Other symptoms, called *particular symptoms,* are those that pertain to any given organ or structure of the body (muscle pain, for instance). They, too, are less important than the general symptoms.

Homeopaths put most weight on what they call *strange, rare, and peculiar symptoms.* As their name implies, they are symptoms that are completely unique to the individual describing them. Describing your hay fever as feeling like a wet blanket covering your face or, conversely, like a dry blaze of fire in your lungs exemplifies strange, rare, and peculiar symptoms. Although allergic rhinitis might be the diagnosis in each case, a homeopath is likely to prescribe quite different remedies.

Finally, it should be noted that an important aspect of homeopathy is the *Law of Cure,* which postulates that symptoms disappear in the reverse order of appearance. In other words, the last symptoms to appear will be the first to disappear with treatment. If you've had many health problems in your life, you might experience symptoms of past problems during the course of your homeopathic treatment. Someone who comes to a homeopath for allergies, for instance, may find that he or she briefly develops symptoms of bronchitis, a previous illness. Slowly but surely, working backward in time, the homeopathic remedy or remedies will restore strength to the vital force and balance to the internal environment.

Treating Allergies Homeopathically

Because treatment is dependent on symptoms, any of the several hundred homeopathic remedies described in Hahnemann's *Materia Medica Pura*, upon which modern homeopathy is based, might be prescribed for your allergies. In addition, a homeopath would work with you to resolve other underlying physical and emotional problems that contribute to your problem. That said, there are some general recommendations for homeopathic remedies that might apply to you.

First and foremost, a homeopath may decide to treat your allergy with a course of minute, diluted doses of the very substance to which you're allergic. For instance, if you are sensitive to ragweed, a homeopath might decide to give you a diluted solution of ragweed (either by mouth or through injection) in order to provoke a less severe but, in the end, quite effective, immune response. Another common remedy used in homeopathy is pollen supplements, which homeopaths prescribe to people with hay fever a few months before hay fever season begins, in order to reduce or prevent reactions once the natural pollen count begins to rise.

In addition, there are several remedies used to treat the symptoms of allergies more indirectly by treating the symptoms. Among them are the following:

FOR RUNNY NOSES, WHEEZING, AND COUGHING

Arsenicum album. Derived from arsenic trioxide—which is deadly in its crude form—this remedy is especially helpful if you suffer from wheezing or have difficulty breathing during your allergy attacks, as well as suffer from severe bouts of sneezing, a strong burning sensation in the nasal passages, and headache. It is often used as a cold remedy, too.

Euphrasia. This remedy, prescribed when symptoms include runny nose, loose cough, and burning tears, is derived from the herb commonly called eyebright. People have used eyebright as an herbal remedy for inflammation of the eyes and sinuses since the Middle Ages.

Sabadilla. Perhaps the most common remedy for hay fever and allergic rhinitis in homeopathy, sabadilla is derived from the cevadilla seed. If a homeopath prescribes this remedy for you, he or she will likely suggest that you try to spend as much time as possible in the fresh air.

FOR HEADACHES (CAUSED BY EXPOSURE TO TOXINS)

Belladonna. Another substance potentially toxic in its crude form, belladonna is derived from a large perennial herb. Its principal active substance is atropine, a central nervous system stimulant. It's especially appropriate for someone whose headaches worsen with exposure to bright light and noise, and when the face feels hot while the hands and feet are cold.

Nux vomica. Derived from the seeds of an evergreen tree native to India and the East Indies, nux vomica is another powerful central nervous system stimulator with a poisonous component, this one strychnine. When an allergen creates a painful headache, causing someone to become irritable, touchy, and anxious, a homeopath is likely to prescribe this remedy.

FOR SKIN IRRITATIONS

Rhus toxicodendron. Derived from poison ivy, this remedy is useful for symptoms that include burning, itching, and fluid-filled skin eruptions that seem to be worse at night. Feelings of restlessness and irritability are also clues that *Rhus toxicodendron* might be a useful remedy for an allergy sufferer.

FOR STOMACH DISTURBANCES

Colocynthis. Derived from the bitter cucumber plant, this homeopathic remedy is indicated if the major symptom is abdominal cramps made worse by eating or drinking.

Ipecac. Long used in orthodox medicine as an emetic (a substance that stimulates vomiting), ipecac is used in minute quantities in homeopathy to cure nausea. Derived from a shrub native to Brazil and the upper part of South America, ipecac is most helpful for people who feel nauseated even after vomiting and whose symptoms tend to come on quickly.

It should be noted that the treatment of any disorder with homeopathy requires ongoing observation and, in some cases, a series of different remedies prescribed on the basis of new, emerging symptoms. Fortunately, the remedies tend to be relatively inexpensive, and once both you and your homeopath better understand your individual makeup, you may be able to administer the remedies yourself at home.

When Dr. Hahnemann first developed homeopathy, modern medicine was in its infancy; the emerging modern pharmacy and operating room were on their way to becoming the mainstays of Western medicine. Today, the World Health Organization estimates that some 500 million people around the world use homeopathy as a treatment for disease, even as high-tech medicine continues to dominate the scene. If you are interested in exploring homeopathy as a treatment option for your allergies or for any illness or condition with which you may suffer, contact one of the organizations listed in *Natural Resources*, page 174, for more information. Next, we explore three different approaches that indirectly help you to better control and cope with allergies: meditation, exercise, and bodywork.

"What is your life, and whence, and where?"

Nikos Kazantzakis

Meditation: Re-establishing Internal Balance

10

*L*ike most Americans, your parents and teachers probably taught you that what happens in your brain (or spirit) has little to do with the rest of your body. Fortunately, a new understanding of the major role that emotions play in our physical lives has begun to emerge, even from the most hard-core modern medical centers. Indeed, we now know that the way we feel, on an emotional and spiritual level, affects everything from the ability of the gastrointestinal tract to digest food properly to the intensity and appropriateness of the immune response. In this chapter, we'll show you ways to harness the wonderful healing, balancing power you hold within your own heart and mind. Although it may take you some time and energy to incorporate meditation and relaxation into your life, it will no doubt be well worth the effort.

Allergies and Stress: A Vicious Cycle

Within every individual who suffers from allergies there exists a direct connection between emotional well-being and susceptibility to allergies. This connection involves stress: the body's response to any stimulus or interference that upsets its normal functioning. Any exciting external circumstance, including the birth of a child, the loss of a job, or falling in love, can be a stress-provoking event. And any internal adjustments your body must make in an effort to keep its chemistry and biology in good working order involve a certain amount of stress. If you fail to eat a proper diet, for instance, you challenge your body to keep itself up and running despite a lack of nutrients. If you have a biochemical imbalance, your body must work extra hard to compensate for it.

Although we hear a great deal about the negative effects of stress, the fact that our body can react in such powerful and effective ways in order to keep its internal environment protected is a very good thing. The most well-known reaction to stress is called the "fight-or-flight" response. An automatic reaction meant to keep us safe from any situation that we perceive of as dangerous, this response prepares us to either stay and fight an enemy (of any kind) or to flee. Such preparation includes raising the heart rate and blood pressure, tensing the muscles, and stimulating all five senses. When we step off a curb only to see a bus heading right for us, for instance, the fight-or-flight response allows us to spring immediately into action and—if we're lucky—avoid making deadly contact with the vehicle.

One branch of the nervous system, called the autonomic nervous system, is particularly important in the fight-or-flight stress response. The autonomic nervous system regulates bodily functions like the heartbeat, intestinal movements, muscular contraction, and other activities of the internal organs. It is divided into two parts that work to balance these activities: the sympathetic nervous system speeds up heart rate, raises blood pressure, and tenses muscles during times of physical or emotional stress, while the parasympathetic nervous system works to slow these processes when the body perceives that the stress has passed. If the sympathetic nervous system stays activated for long periods of time, however, the body becomes exhausted and, recent evidence shows, the immune system disrupted. In order for the body to stay healthy, the sympathetic and parasympathetic systems must work in harmony.

Indeed, the two parts of the autonomic system represent a perfect example of the balance we know of as health. In Chinese medicine, the sympathetic nervous system is the "yang" and the parasympathetic system is the "yin" of the body and its responses. Bringing your body into harmony during and after stressful periods by triggering your parasympathetic nervous system is as important to your health as is reacting immediately, through the sympathetic nervous system, to the perceived threats known as stressors.

Any number of events—physical and emotional—can trigger a fight-or-flight response. One such event is an allergy attack. No doubt you become more anxious when you realize that your skin is breaking out, your eyes are watering, or your stomach is upset in reaction to an allergen. Maybe your palms sweat and your heart rate climbs because you know that the next few minutes (or hours, or days) are likely to involve discomfort, pain, and perhaps unpleasant side effects of medication. Unfortunately, this set of responses does nothing to help you avoid the attack. In fact, it may work to make the attack worse by heightening the symptoms—increasing respiration, for instance, or triggering a rash. In addition, the longer your body remains under stress, the less healthy your immune system will be, which leaves you more vulnerable to future allergy attacks or even to developing new sensitivities.

Helping to Alleviate Your Allergies through Stress Reduction

Is job stress undermining your health? What about your relationships? Your lack of physical activity? Do you live in a hostile environment, either physically or emotionally? If you can answer yes to any of these questions, you might want to consider ways to change your life in order to eliminate or at least alleviate these problems. Chances are, these stressful problems only make it more difficult for you to cope with your allergies or to heal your body so that you can avoid allergy attacks in the future.

In order to break the cycle of stress–allergy attack–more stress–more allergy attacks, you should first try to find a way to reduce the amount of tension and anxiety you feel on a day-to-day basis. Is it possible to change your job? Could you find a way to better relate to your family and friends? Can't you find the time and energy to make exercise a regular part of your life? Although making such fundamental changes may take a great deal of time and commitment on your part, the impact on your general state of fitness and health is likely to be enormous.

In the meantime, there are several other, perhaps more practical, methods of stress reduction available to help you to bring your body back into balance quickly and efficiently during times of stress. In essence, you can learn to counteract the fight-or-flight response by activating your parasympathetic nervous system—your yin to counteract the overactive yang sympathetic nervous system—to attain a more peaceful and relaxed internal harmony. Biofeedback, guided imagery, meditation, and progressive relaxation are just a few of the many techniques known to help release physical and emotional tension. You should try a few different methods, each one for a week or two, before deciding which ones work best for you.

Biofeedback

Biofeedback is a time-tested, scientific method for exploring and utilizing the mind-body connection. It is especially helpful for those people suffering from chronic conditions like allergies. The underlying premise behind biofeedback is that anyone can learn to modify his or her own vital functions—including heart rate, blood pressure, respiration, and muscle tension—by using the mind. In other words, when properly trained, you can learn to slow your respiration and heart rate while reducing anxiety-related itchiness and irritability.

Scientists first developed biofeedback after conducting studies that showed how animals could control bodily functions once thought to be completely automatic by being given a reward or a punishment. Physicians adapted those findings to design ways for humans to control unconscious functions through conscious thought. Although there are several biofeedback methods, they all have three things in common: (1) they measure a physiological function (such as muscle tension); (2) they convert this measurement to an understandable form (a computer-generated graph or chart, a blinking light, mercury levels in a thermometer, etc.); and (3) they feed back this information to the individual.

As with all aspects of health care, it is important that you receive biofeedback training from a qualified practitioner. Generally speaking, that means someone with a firm grasp of both physiology and psychology who has been certified by the Biofeedback Certification Institute of America. See *Natural Resources*, page 174, for more information on how to find a qualified practitioner.

Guided Imagery

Guided imagery is a form of treatment for allergies and other conditions that uses the power of the human mind as its basic weapon. The human imagination—that part of your mind that can picture and sense images and feelings—is one of the most potent health resources available to you. By utilizing the power of the mind, you can help evoke a physical response in your body in order to relax your muscles, stimulate (or depress) your immune system, and reduce tension and anxiety. In fact, guided imagery is now being used to treat any number of conditions in addition to allergies, including chronic back pain, high blood pressure, gastrointestinal disorders, and premenstrual syndrome.

In addition to helping to relax your body, guided imagery also helps to access your emotions. By visualizing your allergy and allergy symptoms as just so many irritating ants that you can step on and destroy, for instance, you may learn to better understand how frustrated and exhausted the symptoms have made you feel, and how powerful and in control of your body you can be if given the chance to break the cycle.

Although it is possible to conduct your own guided imagery session, it is best when learning to have a trained professional develop a program for you and guide you through the steps until they become familiar. Talk to your doctor about finding a qualified therapist for you.

Meditation

Like biofeedback and guided imagery, meditation is a mental exercise that affects body processes. The purpose of meditation for relaxation is to gain control over your thoughts so that you can choose what to focus upon and thus let the stress flow out of your body. Meditation for relaxation requires no special training, and can be done at any time of day and in any comfortable space. All it takes is about 15 minutes of uninterrupted quiet.

Meditation is effective both in reducing general stress and in helping to relax specific groups of muscles made tense by anxiety or worry. When you meditate, you quiet the sympathetic nervous system, thereby reducing the heart rate and state of muscle contraction. In addition to its physical benefits, meditation can help you psychologically by allowing you to focus on the cause of your stress and to find different ways to respond to the challenges you face. Researchers have found that meditation is related to a stronger internal locus of control, greater self-actualization, more positive feelings after encountering a stressful situation, improvement in sleep behavior, and even an increased ability to quit smoking.

There are many good books on meditation available that go into great detail about the proper sitting positions, what to expect, even what to chant if you choose to include chanting in your meditation practice. And there are schools of meditation that train both doctors and lay people in the intricacies of the meditative process. But the basic elements of meditation are very simple, and can be mastered by anyone willing to set aside a few minutes a day.

BASIC MEDITATION EXERCISE

This is a simple meditation exercise that can help you relax and focus your attention away from the things that cause stress in your life. Start by sitting a few minutes—perhaps just 5 to 10—until the practice becomes comfortable to you.

1. Wear comfortable, loose clothing. Sweatpants or shorts and a T-shirt are ideal.
2. Find a quiet place where you will not be disturbed. Try not to sit any place where you might be easily distracted, such as in front of a window.
3. Sit on the floor in a comfortable position. If you can't sit on the floor, sit in a straight-backed chair.
4. Allow your hands to rest on your legs.
5. Lower your gaze so that your eyes are almost, but not quite, closed.
6. Take a deep breath and let it out slowly.
7. The easiest way to begin meditation is to count your breaths. Inhale, count one. Exhale, count two. Inhale, count three. Exhale, count four. Do this to ten, and then start again with one.
8. Sit for about 5 minutes the first week or so (try timing yourself with a kitchen timer so that you don't have to keep track of the time). Gradually increase the time you meditate to 15 to 30 minutes a day.

Progressive Relaxation

Progressive relaxation is a technique used to induce nerve-muscle relaxation. It was developed by Edmund Jacobson, M.D., a physician who designed the technique for nervous hospital patients. It involves tensing one muscle group, then relaxing it, slowly moving from one muscle group to another. The purpose of first contracting the muscles is to teach people to recognize more readily what muscle tension feels like. The idea is to sense more readily when our muscles are tense, then learn to relax them. Progressive relaxation has psychological benefits as well. Studies show that people who practice this method of relaxation over a period of several weeks raise their self-esteem, lessen their vulnerability to depression, and improve their sleep patterns. In other words, progressive relaxation exercises can help you bring your body and mind back into balance.

Usually, a progressive relaxation session begins by tensing then relaxing the muscles of the feet and legs, then moves slowly upward, to the hips, abdomen, lower back, upper back, neck, and arms. After you have more experience with progressive relaxation, you should be able to relax individual muscle groups—the muscles that support the knee or hip joint, for example, or those that control the joints of the fingers. At the start, it may be best to work through your body, from head to foot. The following exercise will help get you started:

PROGRESSIVE RELAXATION EXERCISE

1. Lie on your back on the floor with your knees bent and your feet flat on the floor. Make sure that the small of your back is on the floor so that you do not risk straining the lower back. If you like, support your head with a small pillow.
2. Take a deep breath and tighten the muscles of your feet by clenching your toes.
3. As you relax your feet, exhale. Notice the difference in the way your feet feel.
4. Breathe in again, and tighten the muscles of your calves. Hold the exertion for a few seconds.
5. As you exhale and release your calf muscles, say to yourself, "I feel relaxed."
6. Continue the process, with your knees, thighs, abominal area, chest, arms, shoulders, neck, and face. Each time you tighten and release the muscles, feel yourself sink deeper and deeper into a state of relaxation.
7. When you have finished the process, breathe steadily and deeply for 15 minutes, enjoying the sense of relaxation.
8. Repeat the exercise daily.

No matter what method of relaxation you choose, try to make relaxing a release and a joy rather than a chore. These simple hints are meant to help you find peace and avoid frustration:

Plan to relax. When you know a deadline is coming up, or that a week is going to be particularly busy and stressful, try to schedule some time—even just a few minutes—during each day to perform one of the relaxation methods described above or to simply take a walk to relieve the pressure. Chances are, you'll return to the task at hand feeling rejuvenated and better able to focus your attention. Should you end up having an allergy attack on top of all the rest of your daily stress, you'll be in better shape to cope with it.

Increase your sense of self-esteem and control. Learning that you have power and control over your internal environment and realizing that you can make successful, positive changes in your physical and mental health will automatically raise your self-esteem and give you a new sense of self-confidence. With patience and dedication, these habits may well become a favorite part of your daily routine.

Remember to laugh. Although it may have become a bit of a cliché to say so, laughter truly is one of the best medicines known to man. Humor provides a healthy balance to all the hostility, anxiety, and tension we feel every day. If you can look at the world and yourself with a bit of humor and a touch of whimsy, you'll find that your mind is not as cluttered, your stress is not so great, and your allergy symptoms perhaps less intrusive and debilitating.

If you learn to meditate at the same time that you begin to improve your diet and exercise habits, you're well on your way to taking control of your life, preventing the damage to your sense of self-esteem and general health that allergies can cause, and improving the state of your general health and well-being. In the meantime, the next chapter discusses an aspect of your life that may need some attention: exercise and physical activity.

"There are
some things that
can be sensed
but not explained
in words."

Chinese proverb

11

Exercising for
Health and Fitness

$\mathcal{Y}$ou may wonder why a book on allergies would have a
chapter on exercise. After all, exercise won't clear up your lungs or
realign your immune system. Or will it? The truth is, without regular
exercise, it is impossible for your body to function in balance, harmony, and health. We need physical activity every bit as much as we
need food, oxygen, and water. That's why it's such a shame that so
many people fail to provide their body with regular exercise.

The benefits of physical activity are almost too numerous to mention. In addition to reducing your risk of developing heart disease,
stroke, high blood pressure, some kinds of cancer, and myriad other
diseases, exercise can dramatically improve the *quality* of the life you
live. Exercising on a regular basis will help you look better and
increase your feelings of self-esteem. It will help you release physical

and emotional tension and anxiety, as well as build up your stamina and strength. As each of these benefits becomes evident, you will slowly but surely feel more empowered, more confident, and much less a helpless victim of your allergies.

Although exercising is unlikely to solve your allergic problems, it will certainly help you gain some balance and control over your life and health. Indeed, because exercise is so good for the mind and emotions, it can help stabilize the production of the stress hormones, noradrenaline and epinephrine, so integral to controlling the allergic response. Other body chemicals stimulated by exercise are endorphins and enkephalins, which have mood-elevating effects, helping to reduce stress and alleviate irritability and pain.

Unfortunately, if you're like most Americans, exercise is not a regular part of your life. In fact, the results of a 1994 study performed by the National Center for Health Statistics showed that fewer than 50 percent of Americans perform any kind of exercise on a regular basis. Furthermore, the same study revealed that nearly one third of Americans remain obese—more than 20 percent above a healthy weight. Perhaps you've shied away from physical activity because you're afraid that stressing your body in this way will increase your risk of having an allergy attack. If you have asthma and respiratory symptoms of allergies, exercising—particularly exercising outside—may well have triggered an allergy attack in the past. If so, it is important that you talk to your doctor about finding safe, healthful ways to get your blood pumping and your muscles working so that you can stay well throughout your life.

For most of us, however, our lack of motivation to exercise did not begin because of our allergy symptoms or other physical problems. We may rely on these conditions as excuses, but most everyone—no matter how plagued by allergies or back pain or another chronic illness we are—can add some type of physical activity to our lives. So why don't we? Is it simply because we're lazy and unmotivated? Not entirely. The truth is, there are powerful forces aligned against us on the road to health and fitness. Most of us live in a world driven by very mixed media messages about weight, body image, and lifestyle.

We see rail-thin models advertising fat-laden potato chips and athletes peddling beer. We are prodded to buy time- and physical-energy saving devices like power-driven lawn mowers, snow shovels, and dishwashers. The television set itself beckons to us constantly, urging us to relinquish the physical in favor of the passive

Breaking out of this cycle of inactivity and chronic disease takes time, energy, and commitment. It also requires us to peel back the layers of apathy and of misinformation and frustration about health and fitness that may have built up over the years. Eating a proper diet *will* make you feel better and can be every bit as tasty and enticing as the foods you see advertised. Reading a book or learning a new hobby is *more* relaxing than passively watching television hour after hour.

And as for exercise, it is a positive life-enhancing habit that promotes physical and emotional health and well-being—not a painful, tedious grind. Properly performed on a regular basis, exercise allows you to connect with your physical body in an intimate way. You'll be able to feel your muscles grow stronger, your heart beat harder, and your nervous system throw off the built-up tension and stress of the day. Balance will be restored, balance within your body and balance between you and the rest of the physical world. Every hour we spend in the artificial environment of television, fax machines, stuffy offices, and noisy factories, we get farther from nature and the true role we are meant to play within it.

Exercise and Your Health

In the 1985 edition of the Signet/Mosby *Medical Encyclopedia*, exercise is defined as "any action or skill that exerts the muscles and is performed in order to condition the body, improve health, or maintain fitness." Specifically, exercise helps the body to perform its vital functions in the following ways:

Exercise increases the efficiency of the heart and blood vessels. The cardiovascular system has as its primary function the delivery of oxygen, an element essential to life, to every cell in the body. With regular aerobic exercise (exercise that requires oxygen for energy), the heart and vessels are able to pump more blood and deliver more oxygen and other nutrients to all the muscles of the body. Furthermore, exercise helps keep blood pressure and blood cholesterol at normal levels, thus reducing the risk of heart disease—which remains the nation's number one health problem.

Exercise promotes deep breathing. Oxygen is more vital to our health and well-being than perhaps any other single nutrient or activity. Nevertheless, few of us fully appreciate how important it is to breathe deeply in order to fully expand the lungs and bathe the cells in oxygen-rich blood. That's especially true for those who suffer from respiratory allergies; all too often, we are afraid to really use our lungs and the muscles that surround them even when we're able to.

During vigorous and sustained exercise, an adult breathes about twice as fast as, and much more deeply than, he or she does at rest, increasing air intake from 10 to approximately 20 gallons per minute. By breathing deeply, you allow your lungs to expand and contract deeply and powerfully (especially important if you suffer from respiratory symptoms) as well as help deliver life-enhancing oxygen to every cell in the body.

In addition, according to many Eastern philosophies, the breath is more than a way to physically sustain the life force of cells. It is also the vehicle of the original cosmic energy that has brought everything into being. According to these traditions, how much oxygen we take in, and at what rate, control how deeply energy affects the health of the body and mind.

Exercise stretches and strengthens muscles. Of primary importance to all who want to stay healthy and strong throughout their lives is the development of strong, flexible muscles. Well-conditioned muscles help you perform daily tasks of all sorts (including merely sitting down) with more efficiency and less strain. Good flexibility is thought to protect the muscles against pulls and tears, since short, tight muscles may be more likely to become injured by even moderate activity.

Exercise maintains the body's proper metabolism and weight. With exercise, maintaining a healthy weight comes almost naturally, especially if paired with a relatively sensible diet. First, through regular aerobic exercise, your body learns to burn stored fat more efficiently to use as fuel to meet its increased energy needs. Second, muscle is more metabolically active than fat: the body must burn more calories to feed and nourish muscle tissue than it would to maintain fat. Therefore, the more muscle you have, the more calories you'll burn every day.

Exercise allows the body and the mind to relax. Stress plays a significant role in the development and exacerbation of many allergies. Exercise helps to release both muscular tension and spiritual anxiety. Another benefit of exercise is that certain body chemicals called endorphins, known to dull pain and invoke mild euphoria, are released whenever the body feels pain, including during vigorous exercise when the muscles begin to tire and "burn." Produced in the spinal cord and the brain, endorphins serve as a perfect example of the body's power to return itself to a state of balance and may be the reason that exercise appears to reduce anxiety and stress in those who undertake it on a regular basis.

For all of these reasons—for your general health and to boost your immune system—you should begin to make exercise a part of your daily life. In this chapter, we briefly cover the three categories of exercise necessary to achieve overall fitness: stretching, strengthening, and aerobics. However, it goes far beyond the scope of this chapter to cover any one of these categories in proper depth; each one by itself is the subject of numerous comprehensive books available at your library or bookstore.

If you suffer from chronic allergies, it is important for you to receive proper guidance from your physician, alternative practitioner, or a physical therapist/trainer before you begin to exercise. As careful as we might be to describe exercises properly, nothing beats having someone watch the unique way your muscles work while you exercise, steer you to the exercises that will provide you with the most benefit, then make sure you are performing them efficiently and in good form.

Stretching for Flexibility

Many Americans, even those who consider themselves to be in top physical condition, neglect flexibility. Part of the reason may lie in the noncompetitive nature of stretching. Unlike aerobics and weight training, stretching offers no time or weight limits to beat. Instead, stretching the muscles slowly and steadily to their limit and slightly beyond is an intensely personal effort, one that will bring you closer to truly understanding the unique structure of your own body. Stretching increases the range of motion of a joint, as well as increases the blood supply to the muscle, thereby reducing the chance of injury or strain.

Stretching should always be preceded by a brief warm-up, such as light jogging in place, a few minutes on a stationary bicycle, or a brisk five-minute walk, to increase blood flow to the muscles. When you stretch, you should never jerk or bounce; instead, the movements should be slow and fluid and the position should be held for 10 or 12 seconds at a time. Breathe deeply as you stretch to allow your muscles to enjoy the full benefit of the stretch, as well as to more deeply relax and repair themselves when the position is released. Yoga exercises, which stretch muscles slowly and steadily while bathing the cells in oxygen through deep breathing, are particularly effective in promoting flexibility and increased circulation.

ALLERGY TIP

If you're allergic to ragweed or other plant matter, try to stay inside as much as possible during high-pollen-count days (most local weather stations report the pollen count during their morning broadcasts). If you must go outside, wear an allergy mask and don't participate in strenuous outdoor sports that will cause you to take deep breaths of contaminated air.

Among the stretching exercises designed to increase your flexibility are the following:

Pelvic Tilt. Lie on your back, with knees bent and feet flat on the floor. Hold in your stomach and tighten your buttock muscles. Keeping both your feet and your lower back flat on the floor, lift your hips up off the floor and hold the position for 10 seconds. Release slowly. Repeat.

Lower Back Stretch. Lie on your back, legs straight in front of you. Bend one knee, grasping your lower thigh and keeping the other leg straight. Pull your bent knee toward your chin. Hold that position for 10 seconds. Repeat.

Lower Back Curl. Lying flat on your back, lift one leg in the air to a 45-degree angle, then slowly lower it over the opposite side of your body (probably at about hip level). Keep your lower back and your hips anchored to the floor. Hold the stretch for 10 seconds or so, then repeat on the other side.

Cat Stretch. Get down on all fours, with your hands and your knees on the floor and your back flat like a tabletop. Slowly and gently arch your back, much like a cat does upon awakening from one of its many naps. As you do so, drop your head forward, with your chin close to your chest. Hold the stretch for about 10 seconds, then slowly lift your head and flatten your back. From this position, arch your shoulders back and lift your hips, so that you are in a semi-swayback position; hold for 10 seconds. Then repeat both postures to fully stretch all the muscles of your back.

Shoulders/Upper Back. Raise your right arm and reach down your back as far as you can. At the same time, place your left arm behind your back with your palm facing out and try to reach the fingers of your right hand. Sustain this stretch for 5 to 10 seconds. Repeat with arms reversed.

Chest/Arms. Stand with your left side about arm's length from a wall. Reach out with your left arm and place your left palm on the wall slightly behind you. Keeping your hand in place, turn your body slightly away and to the right. Hold the stretch for 5 to 10 seconds. Repeat facing the other direction and using your right arm.

Calves. Lean forward on the balls of your feet, heels lifted, and bounce very gently 20 times. Then, stand at slightly less than arm's length from a wall. Lean toward the wall, supporting your weight on both hands. Keep your legs straight and your heels on the ground. Hold the stretch for 10 seconds.

Hamstrings. Place one foot about 12 inches in front of the other. Raise the toes of the leading foot in the air. Keeping both knees slightly bent, lean your torso forward as if you were taking a bow. Feel the stretch, for about 10 seconds, in the back and front of your thigh. Reverse the position.

Strengthening Exercises

Overall muscle strength and endurance are critical to general health and fitness; every muscle in the body plays a role in keeping us standing tall, moving smoothly, and sitting properly.

We achieve muscle strength and endurance by applying resistance to normal body motion. The resistance, or load, causes muscles to contract at an increased tension. We add resistance in two ways: through the weight of our own bodies in a series of exercises called calisthenics (sit-ups, push-ups, etc.) and by using adjustable weights.

Because the techniques of calisthenics and weight training are very precise and, if not performed properly, can lead to injury, we suggest that you visit a local gym or YMCA to receive firsthand instruction before you try a program on your own.

A weight-training routine should involve about 30 minutes of slow but constant stress on different muscles of the body using your own body weight (calisthenics), free weights, or strength-training equipment (such as Nautilus). Your exact exercise routine should be formulated with an exercise specialist in a gym, but generally speaking it consists of about a dozen exercises: six for the upper body and six for the lower. Of most importance are exercises designed to firm and tone the large muscles of the body, including the abdomen, shoulders, buttocks, and hip flexors.

The abdominal curl is an especially helpful exercise since it helps to both create a pleasing appearance and strengthen and balance the center of the body. Also known as the sit-up, the abdominal curl is designed to help strengthen your abdominal muscles, which in turn, help keep your back strong and supple. Your abdominals wrap three quarters of the way around your lower back, offering your spine a great deal of support if they themselves are in shape.

Proper form is crucial in performing the abdominal curl. In fact, you will be doing your back more harm than good if you fail to follow the directions outlined below with care. If you experience back pain during or following this exercise, consider obtaining advice about your form from a trained exercise professional at your local YMCA or gym.

THE ABDOMINAL CURL

1. Lie on your back with your knees bent and your feet flat on the floor. Press your lower back into the floor.
2. Tuck your chin close to your chest and place your hands between your thighs.
3. Tighten your abdominal muscles, allowing them to lift your upper body until your shoulders are off the floor.
4. Hold this position for 3 seconds, then slowly return to the original position.
5. Repeat this exercise 10 times.

Please note: Anaerobic exercises, including calisthenics and weight training (with free weights or with Nautilus equipment), are not usually recommended for people with high blood pressure or advanced cardiovascular disease of any type. Such exercises may cause temporary but marked rises in blood pressure. If you suffer from high blood pressure or heart disease, or if you are over 40 and are new to weight training, talk to your physician or alternative practitioner before you begin a program.

Aerobic Exercise

Aerobic exercises are those activities that promote cardiovascular fitness by enhancing the body's ability to deliver large amounts of oxygen to working muscles. Aerobic exercises generally involve working large muscle groups (such leg muscles) for a sustained length of time, generally more than 20 minutes, at a steady, moderate pace. In addition to furthering cardiovascular health, aerobic exercise increases your body's ability to burn fat more efficiently for fuel, a definite boon for people trying to lose excess weight.

There are literally dozens of activities that can provide aerobic benefits if performed over a sustained period of time—at least 20 to 30 minutes—including walking, aerobic dance, cross-country skiing, cycling, swimming, ice skating, running, and jogging. Remember, a prime benefit of exercise is the sense of release and relaxation it offers. You should enjoy this time of your day, not be held prisoner either by the activity itself or by any anxiety you may feel about performing it.

General Guidelines

In the best of all possible worlds, we would get out of bed bright and early, take a few deep breaths, run in place for a few minutes, gently stretch our muscles, then take a brisk walk, a short jog, or play a set of tennis. But for most of us, that is not a reality. Instead, we must work exercise into our lives, slowly but surely making it part of our weekly, if not our daily, routine.

As for strengthening your muscles and increasing your aerobic capabilities, an ideal goal is to exercise about three to five days per week for about 30 minutes. Don't get discouraged if you are not able to meet that schedule at first: every time you move your body, you're doing something positive for your health, even if it's just for 10 extra minutes a day. On the other hand, to really experience a difference in the way you feel about your body and your health, you'll need to make exercise a regular part of your life.

Here are a few tips to get you started on the road to fitness:

Check with your doctor or practitioner. Your first step in starting an exercise program is to consult with your physician or alternative practitioner, especially if you're overweight, over 40, or have any other risk factors for cardiovascular disease. Your health practitioner may recommend that you take a stress test, which measures how your heart and blood vessels are functioning. Both the length of time you are able to exercise and the intensity of activity you are able to endure without becoming exhausted will help your doctor determine a safe exercise routine for you. Furthermore, if your allergies are respiratory in nature or are exacerbated by physical activity, your doctor may be able to work with you to improve your fitness level slowly and carefully.

Consider your allergies. If you suffer from hay fever, then running outside in the spring or fall when pollen counts are high would be counterproductive. If you chose to exercise indoors instead, you'd be much less likely to trigger an allergy attack. If you are feeling ill in any way as a result of your allergies, it makes no sense for you to further stress your body by exercising. Instead, wait until you're feeling better, when your hyperactive immune system has calmed down and allowed your body to return to a normal state of balance.

Start slow. A 1989 study showed that moderate exercise— defined as 30 minutes a day of light activity, such as walking and gardening—is as beneficial to one's health as higher levels of exercise, such as high-impact aerobics and jogging. If you've been inactive for quite some time because you suffer from severe allergies or from exercise-induced asthma, it will take time for your body to adjust. Indeed, moderate exercise is far safer than high-intensity activities for those people who have been sedentary in recent months or years.

Choose activities you enjoy. Perhaps the most important element in the design of your exercise program is choosing activities you will enjoy over the long haul. Think of it this way: if you exercise three times a week for 30 minutes a session, you'll have stair-stepped, jogged, or rowed for about 78 hours—the equivalent of two solid work weeks—at the end of a year.

Set realistic goals. If you've been sedentary for a number of months or years, deciding to train for next month's marathon by running 10 miles every morning would be counterproductive and even dangerous to your health. After failing to meet an unrealistic goal, or straining your body to do so, you'd become frustrated and probably decide not to exercise at all. Instead, set goals you know you can meet, or perhaps ones just out of reach. Achieving them will give you a sense of pride and self-confidence sure to keep you motivated.

Vary your routine. Plan two or three different workout routines in addition to stretching every day. Bicycle one day, walk the next, try a new sport the next. This will cut back on the chances you'll get bored with your exercise program, a prime reason that many of us end up giving up our resolve and go back to being couch potatoes.

Find a support person or group. For most of us, there comes a time when our motivation sags and we lose interest in exercising on a regular basis. When this happens—preferably *before* this happens— enlist a friend or loved one to join you in your fitness quest.

In this chapter, we've stressed the importance of working the muscles in your body, breathing oxygen in to nourish your cells and your brain, and getting your heart to pump harder and more efficiently. In Chapter 12, we'll show you how relaxing under the hands of a skilled professional can bring healing and peace to every part of your body.

"The job of the physician is to entertain the patient while nature heals the disease."

Voltaire

Healing Touch: Bodywork and Massage

12

*Y*our skin is one of your largest and most important organs, covering approximately 12 to 19 square feet and weighing between 5 and 8 pounds, depending upon your height and weight. In addition to forming a protective sheath around your muscles, joints, blood vessels, and internal organs, your skin is also an extremely sensitive and animate structure. A piece of skin about an inch in size contains more than 3 million cells, 100 to 300 sweat glands, 3 feet of blood vessels, and more than 50 nerve endings.

It should come as no surprise, then, that when your skin is touched, the feelings generated reach far below the surface into the very depths of your physical and emotional self. And when stronger pressure is applied, your internal organs—including those involved in producing immune system cells, hormones, and nerve tissue—are affected.

ALLERGY TIP

If you smoke: Quit! In addition to containing a host of potential allergens and carcinogens, smoking depletes the immune system, leaving you more vulnerable to developing not only allergies but a host of other illnesses as well.

For centuries, healers from virtually every culture around the world have used the power of touch as a method of curing illness and relieving pain. In recent decades, massage and other methods of bodywork using the human hands as instruments of health and healing have finally been gaining in popularity and acceptance across the United States as well.

In this chapter, we discuss some of the ways that bodywork techniques can help to heal the body and bring it closer to the ideal state of balance and integrity we know as health. Performed by expert hands, massage is able to:

- Help relax the body by calming the nervous system
- Soothe tense and cramped muscles and joints
- Stimulate circulation of immune system cells
- Trigger the release of endorphins, the body's natural painkillers
- Increase blood flow, helping to remove harmful chemical waste products and allergens from the body
- Help reduce swelling and other symptoms of inflammation
- Release pent-up, potentially toxic emotions through deep breathing and verbal expression during massage
- Bring muscles, bones, joints, connective tissue, and organs back into proper alignment

You have virtually dozens of different bodywork and massage techniques from which to choose. Although the goal of all forms of massage is to return the body to a balanced, healthy state, each technique is slightly different. Following is a brief overview of several different methods available in the United States today.

Therapeutic Massage

The word massage is derived from the Arabic *massa,* which means to stroke. Therapeutic massage, including its offshoot Swedish massage, involves kneading and stroking the skin and applying pressure on tense muscles. Tapping, clapping, or similar percussive hand movements along the spine and muscles may also be employed. The circulation-boosting aspects of massage often help to relieve muscle pain, as well as induce deep relaxation. Massage can be a form of "artificial" exercise that helps blood flow, increases the range of motion of limbs, and helps maintain the suppleness of your body's soft tissues.

Swedish massage, developed about 150 years ago, is the most popular form of massage in the United States at this time. The technique involves five basic strokes:

Effleurage consists of long, gliding strokes from the neck down to the base of the spine or from the shoulder down to the fingertips. Effleurage is designed to acquaint the therapist with his or her subject's body, and vice versa.

Petrissage involves gently lifting muscles up and away from the bones, then rolling and squeezing them, again with a gentle pressure. Petrissage is especially useful for people with allergies whose symptoms include achiness because it tends to increase circulation and clear out toxins from muscle, nerve, and joint tissue.

Friction consists of applying deep, circular movement near joints and other bony areas with thumbs and fingertips. Friction breaks down adhesions, which are knots that result when muscle fibers bind together during the healing process.

Tapotement is a short chopping stroke applied in several different ways: with the edge of the hand, the tips of the fingers, or with a

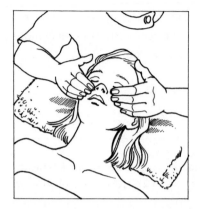 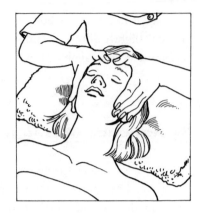

Massage

By massaging certain areas of the face and head,
therapists can help to relieve the headaches and sinus
pain often associated with allergies.

closed fist. Tapotement attempts to release tension and cramping.

Vibration, or shaking, involves the therapist pressing her hands on your back or limbs and rapidly shaking for a few seconds in order to boost circulation and help the muscles to contract more efficiently.

With these five types of strokes, the Swedish therapist will attempt to manipulate all of your muscles, helping you to achieve a new sense of balance and integration. Many health professionals now practice massage, including physical therapists, athletic trainers, and nurses, as well as licensed or certified massage therapists. A visit to a massage therapist typically lasts from 30 to 60 minutes. In most cases, the therapist will ask you to remove your clothing, lie down on a massage table, and drape a sheet over your body. Before she begins the session, the therapist may ask about your medical history and your current emotional and physical state. In some cases, pleasantly scented mineral oils or essential oils may be used during the massage. (If you suffer from skin allergies, make sure to mention your condition to the therapist.)

In addition to Western forms of therapeutic massage, of which there are any number of variations, Eastern techniques of massage also flourish. As discussed in Chapter 5, these include *shiatsu* and *acupressure*, both of which developed out of Oriental medical theory. These forms of massage concentrate on reestablishing the flow of energy in the body so that all organs and tissues receive life-giving nourishment.

The Alexander Technique

Posture—the way we hold our bodies as we stand, sit, and move—has a direct effect on the state of our physical and mental health, or so claimed Frederick Mattias Alexander, a turn-of-the-century Australian Shakespearean actor. Plagued by chronic voice loss, Alexander studied the way he spoke by reciting lines in front of a mirror. What he noticed surprised him: whenever he began to speak, or even thought of speaking, he tended to tense his neck, move his head back and forth, and slightly hunch his back. When he altered these habitual muscular movements, however, he found that his voice returned in full strength.

Based on his own experience, Alexander formulated a theory that the root cause of many disorders, including allergies, may be in the muscular tension that results from holding our bodies in the wrong position over many years. He developed a technique by which practitioners could help subjects "unlearn" faulty movements or postures.

The heart of the Alexander technique consists of allowing your spine to slowly stretch upward to its optimal length by releasing the tension in your neck and lifting your head up so that it sits just above the spine. Whenever you move, you should lead with your head, follow with the spine, and let your body lengthen to its full balanced extent. By doing so, the technique helps to expand the spaces inside the body, including those within the lungs, nasal passages, and gastrointestinal tract. This results in less pressure and congestion. To learn the full details of the technique, however, requires special training.

During a typical Alexander technique session, which can last up to an hour and a half, the practitioner will ask you to either sit, stand, or lie on a table (fully clothed). She will then touch your head, neck, and spine, feeling for any tension or muscular compression, then move your body into alignment, helping you with words and motion to find your correct posture and thus release your joints from any undue pressure. Eventually, over time, you will learn to hold and move your body in a whole new and self-affirming way.

Today, 500 teachers practice the Alexander technique nationwide. To be affiliated with the national professional society—the North American Society of Teachers of the Alexander Technique—a practitioner must have had at least 1,600 hours of training over a three year period.

Rolfing

A biochemist named Ida Rolf, Ph.D., developed this technique, also called structural integration, in the 1970s. According to Dr. Rolf, disease occurs when the body comes out of proper alignment through habitual poor posture and movement. Over time, the fascia (the connective tissue covering muscles and organs) has to compensate and stretch to hold everything in this incorrect and ultimately painful position. Eventually, the fascia becomes more rigid and solid as adhesions, or scarring, occur.

In order to return the body to health and balance, Dr. Rolf suggested that the deep connective tissue be manipulated and stretched back into place. As the fascia returns to its natural position, the blood vessels, muscles, and nerves once out of alignment slowly work themselves back into place. Finally, the body would be remade to conform to its original, balanced design, forming one single vertical line extending from the head and shoulders down into the legs. When this occurs, respiration improves, the body can relax more naturally, muscles and joints work more easily and with more strength, and self-esteem is elevated.

Rolfing, as this technique is called, is not painless. In order to stimulate and realign deep connective tissue, the Rolfer (therapist) must apply some force as he or she massages tissues. It is likely that your first visit to a Rolfer will involve having photos taken of your body in order to assess your posture as you sit and stand. You'll be asked about your medical history, your emotional state, and your current allergy symptoms. You will then lie down on a table or the floor (fully clothed or in your underclothes) while the Rolfer works through your body, kneading your joints and muscles with his or her fingers, knuckles, or elbows. Rolfers receive training at the Rolf Institute in Boulder, Colorado. The course involves two nine-week training sessions, followed by a series of continuing-education classes.

Zero Balancing

Zero Balancing is a simple, yet powerful hands-on bodywork technique, developed by Fritz Frederick Smith, M.D., designed to balance body energy and body structure. Although using a Western scientific base, zero balancing introduces Eastern viewpoints of energy and healing. It works to bring clearer, stronger fields of energy through the body, helping to release tension from both body and mind. This significantly improves physical and mental function, as well as promotes feelings of well-being and optimism in the individual receiving treatment.

A typical zero balancing session takes about 30 minutes. You'll lie on a table, fully clothed, while a practitioner massages and manipulates the joints and soft tissue of your body. The work focuses on the deepest, strongest energy currents in your body. On one level, a session is designed to improve body function by relieving physical pain and mental tension. On a broader level, because of the clarity of energy flow it induces in the body, zero balancing is especially valuable as a tool to help people through periods of life stress, such as a divorce or death in the family. Since we know that allergy attacks can be exacerbated by excess tension, zero balancing provides a helpful adjunct to other treatment for allergies.

Some General Precautions

Although these methods of bodywork and massage are safe for most people, it is important that you follow a few general suggestions before you visit a massage therapist of any kind:

- Receive a thorough medical evaluation of your allergies.
- Massage may not be for you if you suffer from varicose veins, phlebitis, or other blood vessel problems. Vigorous massage could further stress vessels or even dislodge a blood clot.
- Make sure the massage or bodywork therapist you choose is qualified.

You now have had a chance to read about nine different alternative methods of treating your allergies. In Chapter 13, we answer some of the many questions you may have about what you've learned so far.

"Don't deny the

diagnosis,

defy the verdict."

Norman Cousins

Developing an Alternative Plan

13

*Y*ou've now had a chance to read about the many natural alternatives to drug therapy available to help you cope with your allergies and their underlying causes. These options all have a common goal: to bring your body into a natural state of balance so that your immune system can function properly and the rest of your body can work in harmony. They each attempt to teach your body to heal itself, with help only from natural substances, human touch, and common sense.

There are some significant differences in philosophy among these various alternatives, and deciding which alternative is best for you is a highly personal decision, one that may involve investigating several different options before committing to a particular treatment plan. The following ideas about why and how to use and choose an alternative health care method may help you make some decisions about your next step:

Use holistic medicine as a preventive tool. It is never too early to make sure that your body is in balance by following a holistic approach to health, especially when it comes to a chronic disease like allergy. The sooner you take control of your health, the more likely you'll be able to both prevent further allergic reactions and avoid the stress that comes from having a chronic illness—stress that may well trigger or at least exacerbate your allergies and the harm they do to your body on a systemic level.

Invest in some bibliotherapy. A fancy name for learning through reading, bibliotherapy will help you gain a more thorough understanding of the various philosophies of health and disease before you decide how you would like to address your particular medical problem. In *Natural Resources*, page 174, you'll find a list of the most relevant books on allergies and natural medicine from which you can choose should you decide to further expand your knowledge of your condition.

Work with a mainstream physician who is willing to explore options with you. As we move toward the twenty-first century, more and more medicine is bound to include the best of both mainstream and alternative options. If your physician is willing to learn, but does not know much about these options, you can share your resources, and this book, with him or her. If you are currently being treated by a physician who is not open to other philosophies and methods, you may want to consider choosing another doctor more sympathetic with your needs.

Live well and in harmony with the universe. If, after you've read this book, you decide not to pursue an alternative form of medical care, you still should attempt to open your heart and mind to the natural flow of energy, within and outside of your body. Think about the way you live your life on a day-to-day basis: is it truly healthy? Does the food you eat nourish your spirit and your body, or do you end up feeling bloated and grouchy? Are you ever able to relax completely, or do you feel under constant pressure? Are your muscles, tendons, and bones strong and supple, or do you often feel stiff, sore, and achy after performing the mildest of exercise? Consider the way you feel every day, and if you think you could feel better, work to make small, incremental changes in your daily habits—even if you decide to forgo a comprehensive natural medicine approach to your allergies.

I'll devote the rest of this chapter to answering some of the questions my patients with allergies have asked me, not only about their specific problem, but also about the various treatment options described in this book. I hope that the answers provided address some of your own questions and concerns.

Allergies and Alternative Medicine

Q. My allergies come and go—but when they come, they're devastating. I have to take antihistamines by the bottleful, so much that the doctor I'm seeing wants me to start on corticosteroids. Are there alternative therapies that will allow me to quit taking these drugs?

A. All forms of alternative medicine have at least one goal in common: to allow the body to return to its natural state of balance and health. Medications like antihistamines and corticosteroids, on the other hand, work by relieving symptoms without addressing the underlying problem, which is an immune system disruption. It will be very helpful for you to start looking at other options, including tracking down what exactly is causing your allergies, how successfully you might be able to avoid the allergens, and how diet and other lifestyle factors might be influencing your health. In addition, both homeopathy and herbal medicine offer more natural remedies designed to alleviate symptoms such as respiratory distress, skin inflammations and rashes, and gastrointestinal problems. Although you may still need to take standard medication occasionally, you should be able to decrease both the amount and the frequency.

Q. I'm very interested in finding a healthy alternative to drugs and surgery for my asthma and related dermatitis. I'm particularly interested in Ayurvedic medicine, but I've never been a religious person and the emphasis on a spiritual force that helps us heal bothers me.

A. Spirituality is a belief that we are connected to and dependent upon something outside of ourselves, whether that something is nature, each other, or the unknown. It is important to distinguish this from religion, which is a specific belief system that defines and explains that connection. Although Eastern healing systems stem from philosophical and religious beliefs, it is perfectly possible to derive benefits from these systems without subscribing directly to the philosophy. What is important is a belief that you have the power to control your health and your future, and that you can do this by altering the external world (by avoiding toxins as much as possible, changing your diet, exercising, and avoiding stressful situations) and the internal world (by not holding onto negative emotions, by learning to relax, to love, and to play, and by encouraging hope and positive thoughts). Perhaps, through this process, you'll also find a new way to address spirituality in your life.

A Medical Overview

Q. My grandmother had rheumatoid arthritis and now I have allergies. Are the conditions related? Should I worry about my kids?

A. There is some evidence that immune system problems (such as rheumatoid arthritis and allergies) are both hereditary and related to one another. As discussed in Chapter 2, there is much still unknown about the immune system and the way it functions. It could well be that an inherited weakness within that system left you vulnerable to allergies, and that you've passed a similar vulnerability on to your children. Now is the time to start narrowing down your problem by finding out what exactly causes your symptoms and learning ways to prevent them. You also should start to pay careful attention to your children's emotional and intellectual behavior, as well as their physical health, in case they have allergies that cause different—and perhaps more subtle—problems.

Q. I've been working as a seamstress for about eight months. I

ALLERGY TIP

If you are sensitive or allergic to the chemicals found in cleaning products, throw away all bottles, boxes, and cans of the products containing the chemicals that cause your symptoms. Once they're open, it's impossible to seal them tightly enough to keep them from polluting the air. Steer clear of any product that warns it must be used only in a well-ventilated room. Try using baking soda instead of bathroom/kitchen tile cleansers and a vinegar/water solution as a glass cleaner.

---

love my job, but I've developed some skin rashes on my hands and even my shoulders. I've tried some hydrocortisone cream, which works a little, but the rashes always come back. Could I be allergic to something at my job?

A. It's quite possible. Any number of substances could be triggering an allergic reaction. It could be the fabric itself; wool in particular is known to cause allergic reactions in many people. Or it could be some kind of fabric softener or other chemical used to treat the material. Your best bet—short of quitting your job—would be to try to identify the substance causing the problem and avoid that substance if possible. Perhaps you could only work on cutting and sewing cotton and silk pieces if wool or synthetics are problematic for you, for instance. If it appears to be a chemical used in processing the fabric and you have no way of influencing the manufacturer, however, you may need to wear gloves while you work to avoid coming into direct contact with the substance.

Q. What are over-the-counter allergy drugs? Do they work?

A. Man-made drugs, also called pharmaceuticals, are not necessarily "bad for you"; in fact, some drugs may be veritable lifesavers under certain circumstances. Self-described "allergy medications" available over-the-counter are simply less strong versions of prescription antihistamines, decongestives, or corticosteroid creams. They may or may not be effective in alleviating your particular allergy symptoms. In fact, over the long term, they may act only to increase your susceptibility to allergies through a rebound effect. The thing to remember is that all pharmaceuticals—over-the-counter and prescription—usually focus on alleviating symptoms, not on addressing underlying problems. They also tend to take over body functions rather than help the body to work properly on its own. Finally, drugs often produce unpleasant side effects that, in essence, only add to the state of imbalance that caused the original symptoms to occur. Choosing more natural approaches, such as dietary measures, exercise, and herbal remedies, that attempt to restore the body to proper working order while producing a minimum of side effects is often a much safer alternative.

Choosing an Alternative

Q. I want a homeopath to treat my allergies. My mainstream physician, who admits to being able to offer me few solutions, objects strongly. What should I do?

A. That's a delicate question without an easy answer. Many reputable and highly qualified mainstream physicians find it difficult to accept the tenets of homeopathy and other forms of alternative health care because many haven't been "proven" according to strict mainstream criteria. But as more studies confirm that mainstream medicine can offer few if any long-term solutions for chronic conditions like allergies, more mainstream physicians are willing to explore options with their patients. If your doctor refuses, then I might suggest that you find a new mainstream physician, one who is more willing to explore other treatment options with you.

Q. My daughter suffers from allergy-related asthma attacks. We've had to rush her to the hospital three times in the last year because she couldn't breathe. I know in my heart that she's alive today

today thanks to the high-tech medical care she received at the hospital after those events. But I also know that the medicines she's taking can't be good for her body in the long run and would love to explore other, more natural approaches for her. What should I do?

A. There is no doubt that modern medical technology saves lives and can help a patient during an acute crisis. Nevertheless, the effectiveness of modern medicine has its limits, including its typical lack of attention to prevention and its frequent inability to address the root causes of chronic, lifestyle-based conditions like allergies. Fortunately, we are living in a time when high-tech medicine and its holistic counterparts are learning to work in cooperation with one another. Osteopathy is a particularly good example. Osteopaths are medical doctors, with access to, and an affinity for, mainstream medical techniques. Many chiropractors, acupuncturists, and other alternative practitioners also have medical degrees or working relationships with mainstream doctors and health care facilities. Therefore, you'll still have access to the lifesaving diagnostic and medical therapies you feel work for you while investigating holistic options.

Understanding Food Allergies and Dietary Influences

Q. I consume quite a lot of diet soda and frozen foods. I get headaches and stomachaches a lot. Could I be allergic to the preservatives and additives in these foods?

A. Absolutely. These substances are just as apt to cause an allergic reaction as any other and are often ignored by both physicians and people with allergies as possible culprits. Even if you are not directly allergic to a specific additive or preservative, the more of these substances you ingest, the more you overload your immune system and thus leave your body open to additional allergies and sensitivies of all kinds. Generally speaking, then, you should aim to eliminate or at least drastically reduce the number of these substance you consume on a daily basis.

Q. My nutritionist thinks I suffer from "leaky gut" syndrome? What is this, what causes it, and what does it have to do with my allergies?

A. Leaky gut syndrome is a condition in which your digestive tract is more permeable than it should be. In other words, it allows partially digested food particles to pass through the walls of the digestive tract. Once in the bloodstream, these particles trigger an immune system reaction, thereby either directly causing an allergic response to that particular substance or causing the immune system to become overstimulated in general and leaving the body more suspectible to allergies of all kinds. Among the causes of this syndrome are alcohol consumption, use of nonsteroidal antiinflammatory drugs, viral and bacterial infections, vitamin and mineral deficiencies, and candidiasis.

Q. Is it possible to cure allergies through diet alone?

A. Bringing your body into a true state of harmony involves not only addressing nutritional deficiencies or excesses, but also examining your emotional and spiritual state and working to find inner peace. That's why a holistic approach is a good choice for many people suffering from allergies.

Acupuncture and Chinese Medicine

Q. I'm deadly afraid of needles, but I'm ready to try anything that might help relieve my allergies. My brother goes to a traditional Chinese doctor whom he trusts. Should I put my fears aside and go too?

A. Before you decide upon acupuncture, talk to the Chinese health care practitioner about the anxiety you feel about needles. There are many other options within traditional Chinese medicine, including acupressure, massage, herbal treatments, and dietary measures, that you might want to consider.

Q. I have been to an acupuncturist who used a lot of needles and left them in for a long time. My friend went to another acupuncturist who used very few needles, and just stuck them in and out. What is the difference?

A. There are several different systems of acupuncture being practiced in the United States, depending on the acupuncturist's training. Chinese style, as you experienced, tends to use several needles which are retained. Japanese style uses a more gentle stimulation and fewer needles, and French style, favored by many physician-acupuncturists, is somewhere in between. English Five Element style tends to focus on the relationship of emotions to the symptoms, while some others tend to address specific physical symptoms. It is best to discuss the system with the acupuncturist prior to or at the first appointment.

Q. I would try acupuncture, but I'm worried about AIDS. Are acupuncture needles risky?

A. In this era of AIDS awareness, it is highly likely that your acupuncturist is using disposable, single-use acupuncture needles. In addition, all licensed acupuncturists are required to take clean-needle training as part of their examination for licensure. Even so, it is important to ask your prospective acupuncturist if he or she uses disposable needles.

Medicine from India

Q. Ayurvedic medicine seems very elaborate and multilayered. How much do I have to understand before I can start to alleviate my allergy symptoms?

A. Learning about your body from an Ayurvedic perspective is a process, one that may take many years, indeed a lifetime, to go through. An Ayurvedic practitioner will guide you through that process while providing you with practical information about proper diet, exercise, herbal medicine, and meditation techniques. If you follow this advice, you should see positive change in the state of your health relatively quickly, probably within a period of several weeks, depending on your condition.

Q. I don't have a lot of time during the day to both exercise and meditate. Can I do both at the same time with yoga?

A. Yes. Yoga is used as both a form of exercise and a method of attaining a higher state of consciousness through proper breathing and meditation. The beauty of yoga exercise lies in its ability to bring the body into balance through quiet, powerful stretching and the spirit into a more relaxed state through focused breathing and, sometimes, creative visualization.

Herbal Medicine at Work

Q. I'm interested in treating my allergies with herbs. But I also take medication for an ulcer. Can herbs interfere with the drugs I'm taking?

A. Herbs *are* drugs, and yes, if your physician and herbalist do not work together—or are not at least aware of how each is treating you—you could run into some problems with your treatment plan. It's up to you to supply all the people who treat you with a list of any and all medications and remedies you are taking.

Q. Is aromatherapy only used for relaxation, or do the herbs from which oils are derived have physical effects as well?

A. First of all, it's important to realize that relaxation *is* physical. Remember, more and more evidence is surfacing every day that emotion and its effects are present in every cell of the body, especially those of the immune system. The more balanced and in tune you feel, the more balanced and healthy your immune system will be. Second, there is some evidence that therapeutic particles of the original plants enter the body through the nasal passages and the skin and work internally the same way as a dose of herbal medicine by mouth would work. Eucalpytus is a prime example of this principle: inhaling it works directly to open your nasal passages and bronchial tubes.

Q. I'm allergic to penicillin and a variety of antibiotics. Could I be allergic to herbal remedies as well?

A. Absolutely, and you must be sure to inform your herbalist of any and all allergies and sensitivities to drugs and other substances you may have. This information will help him or her provide you with a safe, effective herbal remedy.

Spinal and Cranial Manipulation

Q. Can spinal manipulation, with all of the cracking and pressing it involves, end up hurting rather than helping me?

A. When performed by a trained professional, spinal manipulation will not damage the joints or muscles. In fact, the idea is to bring your spine and other joints back into proper alignment and thus both relieve the aches and pains that occur when your body is out of position and resolve underlying health problems that stem from such a misalignment.

Q. I've been seeing a chiropractor to help relieve my asthma. Frankly, I'm not sure it's helping my asthma, but my blood pressure, which had been on the high side, is now normal. Could there be a connection?

A. Absolutely. Depending on where on the spine your chiropractor is working to alleviate your symptoms, therapy may be helping to reduce your blood pressure in one of two ways. If your chiropractor is concentrating on your neck area, it's likely that he or she is helping to balance the activity of your sympathetic and parasympathetic nervous systems and the effect they have on the function of your heart and blood vessels. The midback area, on the other hand, is connected to kidney function. If your chiropractor has been working on that area, it is likely that your kidneys are producing more urine or your adrenal glands, which sit atop the kidneys, are producing a hormone that helps to lower blood pressure.

Q. What kind of training does a chiropractor usually have?

A. To be certified as a chiropractor, an individual studies at a chiropractic college for a minimum of four years. Training includes all of the basic science and diagnostic skills taught to a medical student, but does not involve surgical or pharmaceutical study. Some chiropractors also learn the fundamentals of nutrition.

Homeopathy and Allergies

Q. I visited a homeopath for the first time last week. After asking me lots of questions about my diet and health problems, he decided to treat my allergies with *Rhus tox*. I understand that this herb comes from the poison ivy plant. I'm quite allergic to poison ivy. Is this dangerous for me?

A. The amount of toxic substance in the homeopathic solution is quite minuscule and thus unlikely to provoke a serious allergic reaction. However, please make sure that the homeopath is aware of your allergy and will keep close watch on your symptoms and side effects.

Q. I'm not sure I understand the way homeopathy works, and what I do know makes me unsure that it really does work, but I have friends who swear by it. Do I have to believe in it for the therapy to work?

A. Having faith that a treatment has the potential to work is certainly helpful, but it is not necessary for you to fully understand homeopathy to reap its benefits. In fact, many homeopaths are unsure themselves exactly how a substance diluted so many times still has the power to heal. Nevertheless, millions of people around the world find relief from a variety of ailments with homeopathy, and you may be able to do so as well.

Meditation: Re-establishing Internal Balance

Q. I have a high-pressure job in computer sales and typically work 10 hours a day and through most weekends. Ever since I started this job my asthma attacks, which used to come and go only infrequently and mildly, have been happening more often and more severely. Is my new job related to my increased asthma problems? Is there something I can do to help myself relax?

A. This is not to say you should switch careers, but you may want to make some adjustments, especially during a time when your asthma seems to be particularly problematic. Is there some way you could sit down for a bit, say 10 minutes every hour? Talk to your practitioner and then your boss to see how you can function in your job without draining your energy and sapping your health.

Q. I know it sounds strange, but every time I try to relax, I get more nervous and anxious. And when I get anxious I start to itch, which seems to bring on a case of hives—which I'm trying to learn to control through meditation and relaxation. I seem to be stuck in a vicious cycle. How can I relax if relaxing makes me nervous? Is there a solution?

A. Take a look at the way you're trying to relax. Although we tend to relate inactivity with relaxation, many people find that activities that stimulate their minds and bodies—such as exercising or working at a hobby—are more helpful in relieving stress than sedentary, passive activities like watching television or trying to force yourself to nap. At the same time, it is important for your general health, as well as for the health of your joints, to try to slow down and quiet your mind on a regular basis. A meditation technique like creative visualization, which does engage the imagination, may be one way for you to both relax and get in closer touch with what makes you such a driven and tense person in the first place.

Q. Every night after I get home from work, I spend 5 or 10 minutes writing down everything that I have to do the next day and all the things that are bothering me. I think it helps me relax, but my wife claims that it only makes my problems seem more important than they are. Who's right?

A. More than likely, you are. A study at Pennsylvania State University showed that people were able to reduce their anxiety levels by setting aside a "worry period" every day. If they started to fret about their problems or future tasks at other times in the day, they forced themselves to postpone it until that period. The organization such a system provided gave the subjects a feeling of control that calmed them down. I'd say you were on the right track.

Exercising for Health and Fitness

Q. My son has what the doctor calls "exercise-induced asthma" related to his allergies. Does that mean he shouldn't play sports?

A. Exercise is one of the most common triggers of asthma in children and young adults. In fact, more than 80 percent of people with asthma wheeze or cough when they exercise, or experience some degree of tightness in the chest. If you are trying to solve your son's problem with natural medicines, which tend to take longer to work than mainstream solutions, your son may need to cut down on his activities—at least until his problem is alleviated. Perhaps, though, you might consider having him use mainstream medications on just those days that he participates in strenuous physical activity. For many children, cromolyn sodium taken a half hour before exercise allows them to play a game of soccer, football, or other sport without becoming ill. Talk to your son's doctor or alternative health care practitioner for more suggestions.

Q. I know I should make exercise a regular part of my life, but I have high blood pressure in addition to my food allergies. Should I exercise or not?

A. Before you start any exercise program, get your doctor's permission. If your blood pressure is sufficiently high, he may recommend that you perform very mild exercises for relatively short periods of time—say, walking at a slow pace for 10 minutes or swimming for half an hour three times a weeks—at least until you build up some cardiovascular and muscular endurance. He will probably recommend that you have a stress test in order to assess the strength of your heart.

Healing Touch: Bodywork and Massage

Q. Much to my surprise, I found myself more relaxed—and far less likely to suffer an allergy attack—when a therapist massaged my feet than when he concentrated on my back or even on my face and sinus area. What's the connection?

A. It sounds as if your therapist is familiar with the concept of "trigger points," or pockets of injured tissue in one part of the body that can cause pain or dysfunction in a different site. Remember, your body works as a unit, and whenever one part of it is injured or unbalanced, another part may well be affected, too. By massaging your feet, your therapist is helping to heal injured tissue or adjust out-of-kilter musculature, thereby returning your body to its natural state of balance and harmony.

In the next chapter, we describe some of the vast resources available to you in your quest for a safer, more effective, and longer-lasting approach to relieving your allergies and bringing your whole body and spirit into a more balanced state.

Natural Resources

....

*M*ore and more Americans are exploring the world of alternative medicine every day, and every day more and more resources become available to answer their questions and meet their growing need for quality health care.

Following are associations that provide information—lists of qualified professionals, pamphlets, videos to explain treatment philosophy, and other supportive material—about each type of alternative approach addressed in this book.

In addition, we also provide a brief bibliography listing some of the many books you can read in order to deepen your interest in and knowledge about alternative medicine.

Acupuncture/Chinese Medicine

American Academy of Medical Acupuncture
(for medical doctors who are acupuncturists)
5870 Wilshire Boulevard
Los Angeles, CA 90036
800-521-AAMA

National Oriental Medicine and Acupuncture Alliance
(non-M.D. acupuncturists)
638 Prospect Avenue
Hartford, CT 06195
203-232-4825

National Commission for the
Certification of Acupuncturists
1424 16th St. NW
Washington, DC 20036
202-232-1404

READING LIST

Beinfeld, Harriet, and Korngold, Efrem. *Between Heaven and Earth: Guide to Chinese Medicine.* New York: Ballantine Books, 1991.

Kaptchuk, Ted. *The Web That Has No Weaver: Understanding Chinese Medicine.* New York: Congdon and Weed, 1992.

Reid, Daniel. *The Complete Book of Chinese Health and Healing.* Boston: Shambala, 1994.

Allergies

American Academy of Environmental Medicine
P.O. Box 16106
Denver, CO 80216
303-622-9755

American Academy of Allergy and Immunology
414 East Wells Street
Milwaukee, WI 53202
414-272-6071
800-822-ASMA

American Lung Association
1740 Broadway
New York, NY 10019
212-245-8000
(or call your local chapter)

Asthma and Allergy Foundation of America
1125 15th Street
Washington, DC 20005
202-466-7643
800-7-ASTHMA

National Institute of Allergy and Infectious Disease
9000 Rockville Place
Bethesda, MD 20205
301-496-2263

READING LIST

McLain, Gary, Ph.D. *The Natural Way of Healing Asthma and Allergies.* New York: Dell, 1995.

Null, Gary, Ph.D. *No More Allergies.* New York, Villard Books, 1992.

Philpott, William H., M.D. *Brain Allergies: The Psychonutrient Connection.* New Canaan, CT: Keats Publishing, 1980.

Randolph, Theron, M.D., and Moss, Ralph, M.D. *An Alternative Approach to Allergies.* New York: Harper-Perennial, 1990.

Aromatherapy

Aromatherapy Institute of Research
P.O. Box 2354
Fair Oaks, CA 95628
916-965-7546

National Association for Holistic Aromatherapy
P.O. Box 17622
Boulder, CO 80308
303-258-3791

READING LIST

Hymann, Daniele. *Aromatherapy: The Complete Guide to Plant and Flower Essences.* New York: Bantam Books, 1991.

Lavabre, Marcel. *Aromatherapy Workbook.* Rochester, VT: Healing Arts Press, 1990.

Rose, Jeanne. *The Aromatherapy Book.* Berkeley, CA: North Atlantic Books, 1992.

Ayurvedic Medicine

Ayurvedic Institute–Dr. Vasant Lad
11311 Menaul NE Suite A
Albuquerque, NM 87112
505-291-9698

Ayurvedic Rehabilitation Center–Loretta Levitz
103 Bennett Street
Brighton, MA 02135
617-782-1727

American School of Ayurvedic Sciences
10025 NE 4th Street
Bellevue, WA 98004
206-453-8022

The College of Maharishi
Ayurveda Health Center
P.O. Box 282
Fairfield, IA 52556
515-472-5866

READING LIST

Chopra, Deepak, M.D. *Ageless Body, Timeless Mind*. New
    York: Harmony Books, 1993. *Perfect Health*, 1991.
    Quantum Healing, 1990.

Frawley, David, O.M.D. *Ayurvedic Healing*. Salt Lake City:
    Morson Publishing, 1990.

Lad, Vasant. *Ayurveda: The Science of Self-Healing*. Santa Fe:
    Lotus Press, 1988.

Biofeedback

Association for Applied Psychophysiology and Biofeedback
Certification Institute of America
10200 West 44th Avenue, Suite 304
Wheat Ridge, CO 80033
303-422-8436

Center for Applied Psychophysiology
Menninger Clinic
P.O. Box 829
Topeka, KS 66601
913-273-7500

READING LIST

Danskin, David G., and Crow, Mark. *Biofeedback: An Introduction and Guide.* Palo Alto, CA: Mayfield Publishing Co., 1981.

Bodywork and Massage

American Massage Therapy Association
820 Davis Street, Suite 100
Evanston, IL 60201
708-864-0123

American Oriental Bodywork Therapy Association
6801 Jericho Turnpike
Syosset, NY 11791
516-364-5533

The Rolf Institute
205 Canyon Boulevard
Boulder, CO 80302
800-530-8875

North American Society of Teachers of the Alexander Technique
P.O. Box 112484
Tacoma,WA 98411
800-473-0620

Zero Balancing Association
P.O. Box 1727
Capitola, CA 95010
408-476-0665

READING LIST

Benjamin, Ben E., Ph.D., and Borden, Gale, M.D. *Listen to Your Pain*. New York: Penguin Books, 1984

Smith, Fritz. *Inner Bridges*. Atlanta: Humanics, Ltd., 1994

Chiropractic and Osteopathy

American Chiropractic Association
1701 Clarendon Boulevard
Arlington, VA 22209
703-276-8800

Cranial Academy
3500 DePauw Boulevard
Indianapolis, IN 46268

International Chiropractors Association
1110 North Glebe Road, Suite 1000
Arlington, VA 22201
800-423-4690

World Chiropractic Alliance
2950 N. Dobson Road, Suite 1
Chandler, AZ 85224
800-347-1011

READING LIST

Coplan-Griffiths, Michael. *Dynamic Chiropractic Today: The Complete and Authoritative Guide to This Major Therapy.* San Francisco: Harper Collins, 1991.

Palmer, Daniel David. *The Chiropractor's Adjuster.* Davenport, IA: Palmer College Press, 1992.

Diet and Nutrition

American College of Nutrition
722 Robert E. Lee Drive
Wilmington, NC 28480

American College of Advancement in Medicine
P.O. Box 3427
Laguna Hills, CA 92654
714-583-7666

READING LIST

Braverman, Eric R., M.D., and Pfeiffer, Carl C., M.D. *The Healing Nutrients Within.* New Canaan, CT: Keats Publishing, Inc., 1987.

Hass, Elson M., M.D. *Staying Healthy with Nutrition.* Berkeley, CA: Celestial Arts Publishing, 1992.

Herbal Medicine

The American Herbalists Guild
P.O. Box 1683
Soquel, CA 95073
408-438-1700

The American Botanical Council
P.O. Box 201660
Austin, TX 78720-1660
512-331-8868

Herb Research Foundation
1007 Pearl Street, Suite 200
Boulder, CO 80302
303-449-2265

The Natural Apothecary
167 Massachusetts Avenue
Arlington, MA 02174
800-841-5523

READING LIST

Castleman, Michael. *The Healing Herbs*. Emmaus, PA: Rodale Press, 1991.

Hoffman, David. *The Herbal Handbook*. Rochester, VT: Healing Arts Press, 1987.

Homeopathy

International Foundation for Homeopathy
2366 Eastlake Avenue
Seattle, WA 98102
206-324-8230

National Center for Homeopathy
801 North Fairfax
Alexandria, VA 22314
703-548-7790

American Institute of Homeopathy
1585 Glencoe
Denver, CO 80220
303-898-5477

READING LIST

Cummings, Stephen, M.D. *Everybody's Guide to Homeopathic Medicines*. Los Angeles: Jeremy P. Tarcher, Inc., 1991.

Lockie, Andrew. *The Family Guide to Homeopathy*. New York: Prentice Hall Press, 1993.

Ullman, Dana. *Discovering Homeopathy: Medicine for the 21st Century*. North Atlantic Books, 1991.

Meditation and Mind/Body Medicine

Institute of Transpersonal Psychology
P.O. Box 4437
Stanford, CA 94305
415-327-2066

Mind-Body Clinic
New England Deaconess Hospital
Harvard Medical School
185 Pilgrim Road
Boston, MA 02215
617-632-9530

Stress Reduction Clinic
University of Massachusetts Medical Center
55 Lake Avenue, North
Worcester, MA 01655
508-856-2656

The Center for Mind-Body Studies
5225 Connecticut Avenue NW
Washington, DC 20015
202-966-7388

READING LIST

Benson, Herbert. *The Relaxation Response*. New York: Outlet Books, Inc., 1993.

Borysenko, Joan. *Mending the Body, Mending the Mind*. New York: Bantam Books, 1988.

Locke, Steven, and Colligan, Douglas. *The Healer Within*. NewYork: Mentor, 1986.

Moyers, Bill. *Healing and the Mind*. New York: Doubleday, 1993.

Yoga

Himalayan Institute of Yoga, Science, and Philosophy
RRI Box 400
Honesdale, PA 18431
800-822-4547

International Association of Yoga Therapists
109 Hillside Avenue
Mill Valley, CA 94941
415-383-4587

READING LIST

Hewitt, James. *The Complete Yoga Book*. New York: Schocken
    Books, 1977.

Alternative Medicine/General Reading

American Association of Naturopathic Physicians
2366 Eastlake Avenue, Suite 322
Seattle, WA 98102
206-323-7610

American Holistic Medical Association
4101 Lake Boone Trail, Suite 201
Raleigh, NC 27607
919-787-5146

READING LIST

Goldberg Group (350 physicians). *Alternative Medicine:
The Definitive Guide.* Puyallap, WA: Future Medicine
Publishing, Inc., 1993.

Micozzi, Marc. *Fundamentals of Complementary and
Alternative Medicine.* United Kingdom: Churchill
Livingstone, 1996.

Monte, Tom, and editors of "EastWest Natural Health."
WorldMedicine: The EastWest Guide to Healing Your Body.
New York: Tarcher/Perigree, 1993.

Murray, Michael, and Pizzorno, Joseph. *Encyclopedia of
Natural Medicine.* Rocklin, CA: Prima Publishing, 1991.

Words and Terms to Remember

....

Acupoints: Acupuncture points throughout the body which correspond to specific organs.

Acupressure: A healing art based on the fundamentals of Chinese medicine in which finger pressure is applied to specific sensitive points on the body.

Acupuncture: A technique used in Chinese medicine that involves the insertion of small needles under the skin to activate the flow of energy within the body.

Aerobic exercise: Physical exercise that relies on oxygen for energy production.

Anaerobic exercise: Exercise that draws upon the muscles' own stores of energy and does not require oxygen, such as weight lifting and isometric exercises.

Antibodies: Protein substances produced by immune system cells that interact with and destroy cells or microbes perceived to be foreign to the body.

Antigens: Substances foreign or perceived to be foreign in the body; result in the production of antibodies.

Anti-inflammatory: Drug designed to reduce swelling, inflammation, and pain. Some common anti-inflammatory drugs include Feldene (piroxicam), Motrin (ibuprofen), and Voltaren (diclofenac sodium).

Autoimmune disease: Disease in which the immune system produces antibodies against the body's own cells, destroying healthy tissue.

Autonomic nervous system: The part of the nervous system responsible for bodily functions such as the heartbeat, blood pressure, digestion. It is divided into two divisions, the sympathetic nervous system and the parasympathetic nervous system.

Biofeedback: A behavior modification therapy in which patients are taught to control bodily functions such as blood pressure through conscious effort.

Carbohydrates: Organic compounds of carbon, hydrogen, and oxygen, which include starches, cellulose, and sugars, and are an important source of energy. All carbohydrates are eventually broken down in the body to glucose, a simple sugar.

Central nervous system: The brain and the spinal cord, which are responsible for the integration of all neurological functions.

Channels: Also called meridians; in traditional Chinese medicine, the invisible pathways of qi on the surface of and within the body.

Chinese medicine: A philosophy and methodology of health and medicine developed in ancient China.

Complementary medicine: The name used to describe the field of medicine that includes acupuncture, nutrition, homeopathy, and other alternatives to mainstream medicine.

Corticosteroids: Hormones produced in the cortex of the adrenal glands; drug versions of these hormones are used to treat inflammation.

CT scan: A tomogram (x-ray image) reconstituted by a computer to depict bone and soft tissues in several planes.

Deficient condition: In traditional Chinese medicine, a disorder resulting from the body's inability to maintain equilibrium.

Detoxification: In Ayurveda, the process of removing toxins from the body.

Doshas: In Ayurvedic medicine, the three basic types of biological humors which determine an individual's constitution.

Endorphins: Natural substances produced by the body which function as natural painkillers.

Epinephrine: Also called adrenaline. A hormone secreted by the adrenal glands that increases the heart rate and constricts blood vessels.

Essential oil: Concentrated, pure aromatic essence extracted from plants.

Excess condition: In traditional Chinese medicine, a condition in which qi, blood, or body fluids are disordered and accumulate in channels or elsewhere in the body.

Fight-or-flight response: The body's response to perceived danger or stress, involving the release of hormones and subsequent rise in heart rate, blood pressure, and muscle tension.

Five Element Theory: In Chinese medicine, a way of looking at the body and the universe that explains the interaction between them.

Holistic: Pertaining to the whole body; holistic treatment of disease is taking into consideration every part of the body to bring the internal environment into balance.

Homeopathic remedy: A remedy that produces symptoms similar to those of the disease and stimulates a reaction in a patient that leads to a cure.

Inflammation: A reaction to injury or infection resulting in redness, heat, swelling, pain, and loss of function in the affected area.

Isometric exercise: Exercise in which pressure is exerted against an immovable object, thus building muscle while keeping joints stationary.

Jinglo: Chinese term for channels or meridians, the network of invisible pathways of qi in the body.

Law of Similars: The principle of "like shall be cured by like" that forms the basis of homeopathy; the proper remedy for a patient's disease is that substance that is capable of producing, in a healthy person, symptoms similar to those from which the patient suffers.

Limbic system: A group of brain structures that influence the endocrine and autonomic motor systems.

Manipulation: Technique used in chiropractic therapy to adjust the spine, joints, and other tissue.

Meridian: In traditional Chinese medicine, one of the fourteen channels in the body through which the energy known as qi runs.

Mobilization: A technique of chiropractic therapy that gently increase the range of movement of a joint.

Moxa: Dried mugwort leaves used in traditional Chinese medicine; placed on the end of needles, then lighted and held near an acupuncture point to warm and tonify qi.

Muscles: Tissues that support the joints and other organs and allow the body to move.

Neurotransmitters: Substances that transmit messages to, from, and within the brain and other body tissues.

Norepinephrine: A hormone secreted by the adrenal gland as a reaction to the "fight-or-flight response" that raises blood pressure and acts to stimulate muscle contraction.

Obesity: The condition in which excess fat has accumulated in the body; usually considered present when a person is 20 percent above the recommended weight for his or her height and age.

Osteopathy: A branch of Western medicine that focuses primarily on the manipulation of the musculoskeletal system while taking a holistic approach to health.

Palpation: Physical examination of the body using hands to feel for abnormalities.

Parasympathetic nervous system: The division of the nervous system that, when stimulated, slows heart rate, lowers blood pressure, and slows breathing.

Pelvic tilt: The body position in which the abdominal muscles are contracted and the buttocks tucked down and under the spine.

Pitta: An Ayurvedic dosha.

Potency: Diluting homeopathic remedies increases their effectiveness, thus giving them their therapeutic value, or potency.

Qi: In traditional Chinese medicine, the life-force or energy of the body and the universe that circulates through the body's channels.

Qi stagnation: Any blockage of energy in the body that interrupts the body's natural functions or the healing process.

Quadriceps: The muscles located in the front of the thighs.

Range of motion: Normal range of movement for each joint, used to measure severity of arthritis; a term used to describe certain exercises.

Risk factor: Condition or behavior that increases one's likelihood of developing a disease or incurring an injury.

Shiatsu: A massage technique developed in Japan and based on the Chinese medical philosophy that believes that disease and pain are caused by blocked qi (energy) along energy pathways in the body. By applying pressure to the blocked meridian, relief from pain and disease may result.

Stress: Any factor, physical or emotional, that threatens the health of the body or otherwise requires a response or change.

Subluxation: In chiropractic, a term used to explain a misalignment of spinal vertebrae.

Succussion: The forceful shaking of liquid homeopathic remedies that allows the permeation of the original substance into the alcohol tincture.

Sympathetic nervous system: The division of the autonomic nervous system responsible for such actions as blood pressure, salivation, and digestion; works in balance with the parasympathetic nervous system.

Symptoms: Observable or internal changes in the mental, emotional, and physical condition of a person; in holistic medicine, symptoms are the external proof of an internal imbalance.

Tao: The course of nature and ways of nature; a Chinese term denoting the universe as an undifferentiated whole.

Tincture: An alcoholic extract of a medicinal substance.

Tonify: In Chinese medicine, to nourish, augment, and invigorate; to add to the supply of qi and to promote the proper functioning and balance in the body.

Toxin: Substance that is harmful or poisonous to the body.

Vata: An Ayurvedic dosha.

Vital force: In homeopathy, the intangible energy that animates all living creatures and mediates their physical, emotional, and intellectual responses to external stress.

Yang organs: In Chinese medicine, the yang organs are hollow or surface organs such as the intestines, stomach, gallbladder, and urinary bladder.

Yin organs: In Chinese medicine, the yin organs are dense, internal organs such as the heart, spleen, liver, lungs, and kidneys.

Yin/Yang: Chinese concept that describes all existence in terms of states or conditions that are different but mutually dependent; traditional Chinese medicine aims to restore balance to these contrasting aspects of the body and mind.

Index

Abdomen in Chinese medicine, 73
Abdominal curl, 143
Achillea millefolium (yarrow), 100
Acidophilus, 25, 50
Acupoints, 74, 188
Acupressure, 74, 75–76, 153, 188
Acupuncture, 11, 68, 74–75, 188. *See also* Chinese medicine
different systems of, 167
needles in, 74–75, 166
resources on, 175
time involved in, 44
Acute illness, 3
Adrenal glands, 24, 169
Adrenaline, 24. *See also* Epinephrine
Aerobic exercise, 144, 188
AIDS (acquired immunodeficiency syndrome), 23, 24, 62, 167
Air cleaner, electronic, 112
Alexander, Frederick Mattias, 153
Alexander technique, 14, 153–154
Allergens, 2, 19, 22, 34

Allergic reactions, 20, 21–24
substances causing, 2
Allergic rhinitis, 1, 29
Allergies
causes and risk factors, 24–26
resources on, 176–177
respiratory, 28–31
skin, 27–28
statistics on, 1
symptoms of, 2, 4–6
treating, 35–37
Alternaria, 29
Alternative medicine, 1–15. *See also specific therapies*
becoming wise consumer in, 45–47
consumer spending in, 7
developing plan in, 159–173
goals of, 161
quiz on, 41–45
resources on, 187
Ama condition, 87, 89
American Academy of Osteopathy, 115
American Allergy Association, 57
American Osteopathic Association, 115
Anaerobic exercise, 188

Anaphylactic shock, 23, 31
Anaphylaxis, 31, 52–53
Anemia, pernicious, 23
Anger, and chronic illness, 5–6
Antacids, 57
Antibiotics, 7, 25, 50, 62
Antibodies, 19, 21, 188
Antigens, 18–19, 19, 189
Antihistamines, 2, 7, 36, 49, 64,
      67, 95, 161
Anti-inflammatory drugs, 36,
      189
Antioxidants, 64
Anti-vata diet, 82
Aroma lamps, 103
Aromatherapy, 12, 13, 95–96,
      100–104, 168–169. See
      also Herbal medicine
   inhalants in, 102–103
   patch test in, 103–104
   resources on, 177
   topical applications in, 103
Arsenicum album, 121
Arthritis
   immune system in, 23–24
   rheumatoid, 23, 162–163
Ashwaganda, 83
Aspergillus, 29
Asthma, 1, 31
Astragalus (Astragalus
      membranaceus), 77, 100
Astragalus membranaceus
      (astragalus), 100
Atopic dermatitis, 27
Autoimmune disorder, 62, 189
Autoimmunity, 23
Automatic reaction, 126
Autonomic nervous system,
      127–128, 189
Avoidance in treating food aller-
      gies, 57
Ayurvedic medicine, 12, 81–92,
      161–162, 167–168
   diagnosis in, 86–87
   goal of, 12
   philosophy in, 84–86
      doshas in, 84–85
      kapha in, 84, 86
      pitta in, 84, 85–86
      prana, 84, 86–87
      vata in, 84, 85
   resources on, 178

   therapy in, 87–92
      diet in, 88–89
      panchakarma in, 87–88
      yoga in, 89–92

Bacteria, 18
Baker's yeast, 62
Balanced breathing, 91–92
Basil, 83
Bath oils, 103
B cells, 19, 21, 64
Belladonna, 122
Beta-carotene, 63, 64
Bibliotherapy, 160
Biofeedback, 14, 128–129, 189
   resources on, 179
Biofeedback Certification Insti-
      tute of America, 129
Blood pressure, 172
Blue dragon, 77
Bodywork, 14–15, 172–173.
      See also Massage
   and functioning of adrenal
      glands, 24
   resources on, 180
   techniques in, 150
Breath, shortness of, and
      chronic illness, 5
Breathing, benefits of exercise
      in, 138
Breathing exercises
   in Ayurvedic medicine, 91–92
   in Chinese medicine, 77–78
   in osteopathy, 115
B vitamins, 64–65

Calamus, 83
Calves stretch, 142
Candida albicans, 26, 61, 62
Candidiasis, 26
Capsaicin, 99
Capsicum minimum (cayenne),
      99
Capsules, 98
Carbohydrates, 61, 189
Cardamon, 77
Cat stretch, 141
Cayenne (Capsicum minimum),
      99
Central nervous system, 189

Chamomile, 104
Channels, 189
Chest/arms stretch, 141
Chinese medicine, 11, 67–74,
     76–78, 189. *See also*
     Acupuncture
  acupuncture in, 68, 74–75
  diagnosis and treatment in,
     76–77
  herbs in, 76–77
  medical history in, 73
  philosophy in, 69–71
     climatic conditions, 70
     qi, 70–71, 76
     yin/yang in, 69–70
  physical examination in,
     73–74
  qi-gong exercises in, 77–78
  resources on, 175
  shiatsu in, 76
Chiropractic, 13. *See also*
     Osteopathy
  diagnosis in, 110–111
  finding qualified practitioner,
     111–112
  and functioning of adrenal
     glands, 24
  resources on, 181
  techniques in, 109–110
  therapy in, 111
  time involved in, 44, 111
Chiropractor
  certification of, 169
  finding qualified, 111–112
Chopra, Deepak, 89
Chronic illness, challenge of, 3–6
Chyavan Prash, 83
Circulation-sex energy, 74
Cleaning products, sensitivity
     to, 163
Collagen, 23
Colocynthis, 122–123
Complementary medicine, 189
Contact dermatitis, 27
Corticosteroids, 7, 36, 161, 189
Cosmetics, sensitivity to, 88
Cranial manipulation, 114
Cranial osteopathy, 13,
     107–108, 113
Craniosacral therapy, 107–108
Creative visualization, 171
Crohn's disease, 62

Cromolyn sodium, 36, 172
CT scan, 190
Cumulative reactions, 52
Cure, law of, 120

Damp heat, 68
Dander, allergies to, 29
Decongestants, 36, 67, 95
Deficient condition, 190
Depression, 32
  and chronic illness, 6
Dermatitis
  atopic, 27
  contact, 27
Dermatologist, 33
Dermatology, 33
Detoxication, 190
Diagnosis
  in Ayurvedic medicine, 86–87
  in Chinese medicine, 72–78
  in chiropractic, 110–111
  importance of obtaining
     accurate, 45
  in osteopathy, 113–114
Dichromates, 27
Diet, 41, 43
  and allergies, 25–26
  anti-vata, 82
  in Ayurvedic medicine, 88–89
  elimination challenge, 54–56
  and improving eating habits,
     58–63
  influence on food allergies,
     10–11, 165
  in maintaining healthy
     weight, 59–62
  nutritional supplements in,
     50, 63–65
  in osteopathy, 115
  planning healthy, 56
  resources on, 182
  rotation, 57–58
Diet diary, 50
Diffusers, 103
Doshas, 12, 190
Dust, allergies to, 29

Eating habits, improving, 58–63
Echinacea *(Echinacea angusti-
     folia)*, 100

Echinacea angustifolia (echinacea), 100
Eczema, 27
Effleurage in Swedish massage, 151
Electronic air cleaner, 112
Elimination challenge diet, 54–56
Emotional component of health, 8–9, 125
Emotional stress, and allergies, 26
Endocrine system, 24
Endorphins, 136, 190
Enkephalins, 136
Eosinophils, 22
Ephedra, 77
Epinephrine, 24, 136, 190
Essential cell, 190
Essential oils in aromatherapy, 13, 97, 101–103
Ethylenediamine, 27
Eucalyptus, 168
Eucalyptus oil, 101–102, 105
Euphrasia, 122
Excess condition, 190
Exercise, 14, 135–146
    aerobic, 144
    basic meditation, 131
    benefits of, 51, 135–136, 137–139, 172
    definition of, 137
    flexibility, 140–142
    guidelines for, 144–146
    progressive relaxation, 132–133
    qi-gong, 11, 77–78
    strengthening, 142–143
    yoga in, 89–92, 167–168
Extracts, 98
Eyebright, 122

Facial saunas, 103
Fatigue, and chronic illness, 4
Fight-or-flight response, 24, 126, 128, 190
Five Element Theory, 72, 190
Fixed reactions, 52
Flavonoids, 63
Flexibility, exercising for, 140–142

Food addiction, 53
Food allergies, 43, 49–65
    anaphylaxis in, 52–53
    cumulative reactions in, 52
    dietary influences on, 165
    diet in, 25–26
    and entertaining, 71
    fixed reactions in, 52
    gastrointestinal distress in, 32
    headaches in, 31
    importance of reading labels in, 53, 56
    and improving eating habits, 58–63
    influence of diet on, 10–11
    need to read labels, 28
    nutritional supplements in, 63–65
    problems in diagnosing, 53–57
    RAST testing for, 34
    symptoms in, 10–11, 49, 51
    treating, 57–58
    variable reactions in, 52
Free radicals, 64
Friction in Swedish massage, 151
Fungi, 18

Gamma globulin, 22
Ganoderma mushroom, 77
Gastrointestinal distress, 32
Gattefossé, René-Maurice, 101
Genetics, and allergies, 24–25
Ghee, 83
Gluten, 52
Goldenseal *(Hydrastis canadensis)*, 99
Gotu koa, 83
Guided imagery, 14, 129–130

Hahnemann, Samuel, 14, 117, 118–119, 121, 123
Hamstrings stretch, 142
Hay fever, 1, 29
Headaches, 31
Health, emotional component of, 8–9
Health maintenance organizations, 117–118

Heart protector, 72
Hepatitis, 22
Herbal medicine, 11, 12–13,
    95–105, 168–169. *See
    also* Aromatherapy
    Chinese, 76–77
    forms of herbs in, 98
    in reducing inflammation,
        99–100
    in reducing mucus accumu-
        lation, 99
    resources on, 183
    in strengthening immune
        system, 100
High-efficiency particulate air
    (HEPA) filters, 112
High-velocity thrusts, 111
Hippocrates, 113
Histamines, 22, 23
Hives, 27–28, 171
Holistic medicine, 190
    benefits of, 6–9
    as preventive tool, 160
    time involved in, 44
    and treatment of allergies, 6
Holistic practitioner
    establishing relationship
        between mainstream
        practitioner and, 47
    interviewing, 46
    investigating credentials of, 46
    preparing for first
        appointment with, 46–47
Homeopathy, 13–14, 44, 115,
    117–123, 164, 170
    philosophy in, 118–119
    remedies in, 119–123, 190
    resources on, 184
    symptoms in, 120
Hormodendrum, 29
Hormones, 24
Hydrastis canadensis
    (goldenseal), 99

Imagery, guided, 129–130
Immune deficiency, 23
Immune responses, 19, 21
Immune system, 2, 18–26
    effect of stress on, 2
    herbs used to strengthen, 100
    mind/body approach to, 8

Immunity, 18
Immunoglobulin A (IgA), 21, 63,
    89
Immunoglobulin D (IgD), 22
Immunoglobulin E (IgE), 21, 22,
    23, 34
Immunoglobulin G (IgG), 22
    in RAST test, 34, 50
Immunoglobulin M (IgM), 21
Immunoglobulins, 19, 21–23, 64
Immunologist, 33
Immunology, 33
Immunosuppressants, 26
Immunotherapy, 36
Infinitesimals, Law of, 119
Inflammation, 190
    herbs used in treating,
        99–100
Inhalants, essential oils as,
    102–103
Ipecac, 123
Irritability, 32
Irritable bowel syndrome, 68
Isometric exercise, 191
Isometrics, 77
Isothenics, 77

Jade screen, 76
Jinglo, 191

Kapha, 12, 84, 86
Kinins, 23

Lactose intolerance, 53–54
Lavender *(Lavandula officinalis)*,
    105
Lavender oil, 101
Law of Cure, 120
Law of Infinitesimals, 119
Law of Similars, 119, 191
Leaky gut syndrome, 166
Lethargy, 32
Leukotrines, 23
Limbic system, 191
Lower back curl, 141
Lower back stretch, 141
Lunar pranayama, 82
Lymphocytes, 18

Magnolia, 76
Mainstream medicine
    diagnosis of allergies in,
        32–35
    and evaluation of condition,
        10
    and treatment of allergies, 6
    establishing relationship
        between holistic practi-
        tioner and, 47, 160, 164
Manipulation, 191
Massage, 14–15, 172–173. *See
    also* Bodywork
    Alexander technique in, 14,
        153–154
    precautions in, 156
    resources on, 180
    Rolfing in, 14–15, 154–155
    shiatsu in, 76
    therapeutic, 151–153
    zero balancing in, 155
Massage oils, 103
Materia Medica Pura
    (Hahnemann), 121
Mediators, 22
Medical history
    in aromatherapy, 97
    in Chinese medicine, 73
    in chiropractic, 110
    in diagnosing allergies, 34
Medicines, overstimulation by,
    25
Meditation, 14, 125–133, 130,
    170–171
    basic exercise in, 131
    resources on, 185
Memory cells, 21
Mental health, 41–42, 43–44
Meridians, 70, 71, 73, 75, 191
Metabolism, benefits of
    exercise for, 139
Mind/body medicine, resources
    on, 185
Mites, 29
Mobilization, 191
Mold, allergies to, 29
Monosodium glutamate (MSG),
    31, 52
Mood disturbances, 32
Mother tincture, 119
Moxa, 68, 74, 75, 191
Moxibustion, 75

Mucus accumulation, herbs
    used in treating, 99
Multiple sclerosis, 62
Muscles, 191
    benefits of exercise for, 138

National Academy of Allergy
    and Immunology, 57
National Institutes of Health,
    establishment of Office
    of Alternative Medicine
    in, 6, 39–40
Nautilus equipment, 142, 143
Needles in acupuncture, 11,
    74–75, 166
Netti pot, 82–83
Neurological examination in chi-
    ropractic, 110
Neurotransmitters, 191
Niacin, 65
Nickel compounds, 27
Noradrenaline, 136. *See also*
    Norepinephrine
Norepinephrine, 191. *See also*
    Noradrenaline
North American Society of
    Teachers of the Alexander
    Technique, 154
Novocain, 27
Nutrition. *See* Diet
Nutritional deficiency, 25
Nutritional supplements, 50,
    63–65
Nux vomica, 122

Obesity, 192
Office of Alternative Medicine,
    establishment of, in
    National Institutes of
    Health, 6, 39–40
Ointments, 98
Orthodox medicine, 118
Osteopaths
    finding qualified, 115
    training for, 13
Osteopathy, 13, 107–108,
    112–115, 165, 192. *See
    also* Chiropractic

Osteopathy *(continued)*
 diagnosis in, 113–114
 finding qualified practitioner
  in, 115
 resources on, 181
 therapy in, 114–115
Otorhinolaryngologist, 33
Otorhinolaryngology, 33
Over-the-counter allergy drugs,
 163–164

Pain, and chronic illness, 5
Palmer, Daniel David, 109
Palpation, 192
Panchakarma, 87–88
Paraphenylenediamine, 27
Parasympathetic nervous sys-
 tem, 127, 128, 192
Passive manipulation, 111
Patch test in aromatherapy,
 103–104
Pelvic tilt, 141, 192
Pe Min Wan, 68
Penicillin, 27, 31
Penicillium, 29
Perfect Health (Chopra), 89
Pernicious anemia, 23
Petrissage in Swedish
 massage, 151
Pharmaceuticals, 163–164
Physical aspects of health care,
 41, 42–43
Physical examination
 in Chinese medicine, 73–74
 in chiropractic, 110–111
 in osteopathy, 113–114
Pinellia, 77
Pitta, 82, 192
Plasma cells, 19
Poison ivy, oak, and sumac, 27
Pollen count, 140
Poria cocos, 77
Posture, qi-gong, 78
Posture correction, in osteopa-
 thy, 115
Potency, 192
Poultices, 98, 103
Prana, 12, 86–87
Pranayama, 91–92
Processed foods, 53

Progressive biofeedback, 14
Progressive relaxation, 131–132
 exercise in, 132–133
Prostaglandins, 23
Protozoa, 18
Pueraria, 76
Pulse
 in Ayurvedic medicine, 86–87
 in Chinese medicine, 73
Purple cornflower, 100

Qi, 11, 70–71, 75, 76, 192
Qi-gong exercices, 11, 77–78
Qi stagnation, 192
Quadriceps, 192

Radioallergosorbent tests
 (RAST) in diagnosing
 allergies, 34, 49–50, 54
Range of motion, 192
Red sage *(Salvia officinalis)*, 99
Rehmannia, 77
Relaxation
 benefits of exercise for, 139
 in osteopathy, 114
 progressive, 131–132
Respiratory allergies, 28–31
Rheumatoid arthritis, 23, 62,
 162–163
Rheumatologist, 33
Rheumatology, 33
Rhizopus, 29
Rhus toxicodendron, 122
Risk factors for allergies, 24–26,
 192
Rolf, Ida, 154
Rolfing, 14, 154–155
Rosemary oil *(Rosmarinus
 officinalis)*, 105
Rotation diet, 50, 57–58
Rubber compounds, 27

Sabadilla, 122
Salvia officinalis (red sage), 99
Satvajaya, 88
Sclerosis, multiple, 62
Selenium, 64
Shiatsu, 76, 153, 192
Shock, anaphylactic, 23, 31

Shoulders/upper back stretch, 141
Similars, Law of, 119, 191
Skin, 149
Skin allergies, 27–28
Skin tests in diagnosing allergies, 34, 49, 54, 67, 81
Skull, 108
Smith, Fritz Frederick, 155
Spinal and cranial manipulation, 13, 107–115, 169
Spinal cord, 108
Spirituality, 162
Still, Andrew Taylor, 112–113
Strengthening exercises, 142–143
Streptomycin, 27
Stress, 192
    and chronic illness, 5
    effect of, on immune system, 2
    emotional, 26
    management of, 127–128, 171–172
    role of, in allergies, 126–127
Subluxation, 111, 192
Succussion, 119, 193
Sugar, 61
Sun Salutation, 89–92
Swedish massage, basic strokes in, 151–152
Sympathetic nervous system, 127–128, 193
Symptoms, 193

Tablets, 98
Tai yin meridian, 75
Tangerine peel, 77
Tao, 69, 193
Tapotement in Swedish massage, 151–152
T cells, 19
T-helper cells, 23
Therapeutic massage, 151–153
Tinctures, 98, 193
Tongue
    in Ayurvedic medicine, 82, 87
    in Chinese medicine, 73
Tonification, 88, 193
Toxins, 21, 193
    overexposure to, 25

Trigger points, 173
Tyramine, 31

Urticaria, 27–28

Vata, 82, 193
Vertebrae, 108–109, 111
Vibration in Swedish massage, 152
Viruses, 18
Visualization, creative, 171
Vital force, 118, 193
Vitamin A, 63
Vitamin C, 63, 64
Vitamin E, 64

Weight control, 59–62
    benefits of exercise for, 139
Western forms of therapeutic massage, 152–153
White blood cells, 18, 22
Whole herbs, 98
World Health Organization, 123
Worsley, J. R., 72

Xanthium, 68, 76

Yang ming meridian, 75
Yang organs, 193
Yarrow (Achillea millefolium), 100
Yeast, 61
    allergy to, 11
    overgrowth, 25
Yeast infections, 50, 62
Yellow Emperor's Canon of Internal Medicine, 69
Yellow root, 99
Yin organs, 193
Yin/yang, 11, 69–70, 127, 193
Yoga, 167–168
    resources on, 186
    Sun Salutation in, 89–92

Zero balancing, 155
Zinc, 63

About the Authors

Glenn S. Rothfeld, M.D.

Glenn S. Rothfeld, M.D., is founder and Medical Director of Spectrum Medical Arts in Arlington, Massachusetts, a comprehensive primary care center blending orthodox and complementary medical styles. He holds one of the nation's first Master's Degrees in acupuncture and is director of Western Medical Curriculum at the New England School of Acupuncture. He is also Clinical Instructor at Tufts University School of Medicine, where he teaches a popular course in Natural Medicine.

Suzanne LeVert

Suzanne LeVert is a writer who specializes in health and medical subjects. Her recent titles include A Woman Doctor's Guide to Menopause, Parkinson's Disease: A Complete Guide for Patients and Caregivers, *and* If It Runs in the Family: Hypertension and Diabetes. *She lives in Boston, Massachusetts.*